The SLP's IEP Companion

Third Edition

Carolyn C. Wilson

Janet R. Lanza

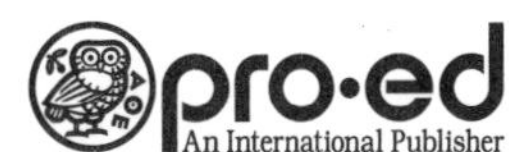

8700 Shoal Creek Boulevard
Austin, Texas 78757-6897
800/897-3202 Fax 800/397-7633
www.proedinc.com

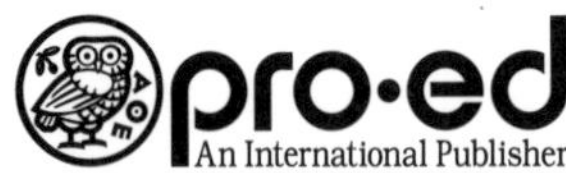

© 2018, 2005, 1992 by PRO-ED, Inc.
8700 Shoal Creek Boulevard
Austin, Texas 78757-6897
800/897-3202 Fax 800/397-7633
www.proedinc.com

Library of Congress Cataloging-in-Publication Data

Names: Wilson, Carolyn C., 1941- author. | Lanza, Janet R., author.
Title: The SLP's IEP companion / Carolyn C. Wilson, Janet R. Lanza.
Description: Third edition. | Austin, Texas : PRO-ED, 2018. | Includes bibliographical references.
Identifiers: LCCN 2017031900 (print) | LCCN 2017037041 (e-book) | ISBN 9781416410874 (e-book PDF) | ISBN 9781416410867 (print)
Subjects: LCSH: Speech therapy for children. | Communicative disorders in children—Treatment. | Interpersonal communication--Study and teaching.
Classification: LCC LB3454 (e-book) | LCC LB3454 .W55 2018 (print) | DDC 371.91/42—dc23
LC record available at https://lccn.loc.gov/2017031900

Art Director: Jason Crosier
Designer: Tom de Lorenzo
This book was designed in Universe, Myriad Pro, and Formata.

Printed in the United States of America

3 4 5 6 7 8 9 10 11 12 27 26 25 24 23 22 21 20 19 18

Dedication

Over the years, we have received much support from family, friends, colleagues, and mentors, which has enabled us to pass on to others some of the care that we have received. We have learned that those who struggle with communication problems need a special kind of care and concern, as well as information, if they are to grow to become communicators. Our profession has given us countless opportunities to pass on such care and information to our students and their families. Our desire for *The SLP's IEP Companion, Third Edition* is that it will aid in the development of intervention programs by the SLPs who use it and dedicate their own expertise and care to their students and patients. Our sincere dedication of this book is to that objective.

Carolyn and Janet

Dedication

Contents

Foreword

Some things last longer than others. *The SLP's IEP Companion,* authored by Carolyn Wilson and Janet Lanza, has shown exceptional staying power. Throughout the almost 30 years of publication of this book, the authors have shared the ability of expert clinicians to follow new clinical evidence and current trends in special education and speech and language pathology and incorporate them into their work. This new edition of the book follows this pattern and provides an excellent guide for identifying learning objectives and outcomes and implementing intervention objectives for clinicians in our field. With each edition the scope of the content of the work has been expanded and updated to reflect new clinical evidence. This edition adds new yearly goals, short-term goals, objectives, and examples to an already extensive range. There was also a complete revision of the literacy units for reading and writing. In addition, the prior and the newest objectives have been tied to the Common Core State Standards. It is an honor for me to introduce my fellow SLPs to the newest edition of a valuable and trusted companion.

Elisabeth H. Wiig, PhD

Acknowledgments

We were fortunate to have received valuable suggestions and guidance from colleagues. Jeannie Evans was with us from the beginning and coauthored this work through all of the previous revisions. Valerie Johnston, MS, CCC-SLP, wrote the individual objectives for fluency and provided guidance to us in writing the intervention objectives. Sherrie Wilson, advanced placement reading specialist, reviewed the units on reading, writing, critical thinking, and study skills. Lynn Flahive, MS, CCC-SLP (Texas Christian University), reviewed the speech production unit and provided the research basis for the decision to omit the oral-motor unit. Colleagues in the Davies School of Communication Sciences and Disorders at Texas Christian University were generous in loaning us books and reference materials. Finally, our families receive our appreciation and love. They supported us even when we were at the computer for hours on end. Our children, Allison Lanza and Scott Wilson, offered invaluable technical help. Our families encouraged us until the last word was written.

Introduction

The SLP's IEP Companion, Third Edition is a resource for speech–language pathologists (SLPs) for use in planning individualized intervention and writing Individualized Education Program (IEP) goals for children and adolescents through Grade 12. The scope covers students and clients from age 3 months to adult. The yearly goals and objectives of *The SLP's IEP Companion* are correlated to the Common Core State Standards (CCSS) (Common Core State Standards Initiative, 2010). These standards are research based and based on state education standards. They are a tool to help SLPs develop interventions relevant to students' current and future educational needs. The third edition has been updated to incorporate both the feedback of SLPs who have used the text and the professional experience of the authors. SLPs working in schools, clinics, or other settings, such as hospitals or private practice, will find this manual invaluable when planning intervention.

In 1983, LinguiSystems published the original version of this manual as *SCOR: Sequential Communication Objectives for Remediation* (Barton, Lanza, & Wilson, 1983). It was conceived as a practical solution to challenges the authors faced as SLPs in a local school district. With the passage in 1975 of Public Law 94-142, the Education for All Handicapped Children Act (amended in 1997 as the Individuals With Disabilities Education Act, or IDEA), SLPs were faced with the task of creating individual developmental yearly goals and objectives for each student as a part of his or her IEP.

The IEP Companion: Communication Goals for Therapy in and out of the Classroom, published by LinguiSystems (C. Wilson, Lanza, & Evans, 1992), was the original edition of *The SLP's IEP Companion*. LinguiSystems published a second edition, titled *The SLP's IEP Companion*, in 2005. Four new units were added at that time: Critical Thinking, Organization and Study Skills, Literacy: Reading, and Literacy: Writing. The appendixes grew to include First Words, Word Lists, Visual Organizers, Purposes for Writing, Writing Frames, and Fluency Facilitators. *The SLP's IEP Companion, Second Edition* was subsequently acquired by PRO-ED, Inc. This newest edition is the third edition, and it includes important updates and improvements.

Changes to the Third Edition

The SLP's IEP Companion presents goals and objectives in a scope and sequence that is broad enough to apply to many types of speech and language disorders, as well as a wide range of ages, yet flexible enough to be used with many different programs and clinical perspectives. The sequences of objectives are organized for easy access for SLPs when constructing programs or sequences of therapy. Because the objectives are arranged in developmental order, they can provide progress points when other structured programs are being used. It is expected that the objectives will be adapted to meet the needs of the students or clients served.

The following changes have been made in the third edition.

Common Core State Standards Correlated With Goals and Objectives

"The CCSS were built on existing state standards using specific criteria and considerations. They are research-based and include integration of best practices and education research from throughout the world" (ASHA, n.d.). The mission of the CCSS is to provide an understanding of what students are expected to learn. The standards are designed to reflect the knowledge and skills needed for success in college and careers.

The 11 units in *The SLP's IEP Companion* are divided into more than 70 sections, more than two thirds of which contain goals and objectives that correlate with the CCSS. The correlations are an effective way to support students' regular and special education goals. This addition is invaluable for SLPs who desire to coordinate interventions with the school curriculum.

Refer to Appendix H to see *The SLP's IEP Companion* "Correlation With Common Core State Standards." To see the full text of the standards, go to www.corestandards.org. Individual standards can be searched online by entering the code for a standard or even the last few numbers or letters of the code.

New Objectives

There are more than 100 new objectives, with the total objectives exceeding 1,100. Some objectives were added as they tied to the CCSS. Others were added to expand the lower level sections for the youngest children and the higher level objectives for more advanced students, especially in the area of writing.

New Examples

Examples of ways to teach each objective have been added. Each objective is matched with an easy-to-follow educational or therapeutic activity and a specific example of what to do or say.

New Short-Term Goals

Many sections within the units are divided into smaller parts according to the short-term goals that support the yearly goal. The "Short-Term Goal" headings make it easy to scan through objectives and examples when planning intervention.

Literacy: Reading Unit

Objectives in the new unit Literacy: Reading correlate with more standards from the CCSS than all other units in *The SLP's IEP Companion*. The objectives in the Phonological Awareness section were written to match the CCSS for PreK–Grade 1. Seven new objectives were added to Reading Literature and Reading Informational Text.

Literacy: Writing Unit

Twelve new objectives, many correlated with the CCSS, were added to the Literacy: Writing unit. A new visual organizer and characterization map were added to Appendix C for use with the Literacy: Writing unit.

Omission of the Oral Motor Unit

The Oral Motor unit from the 2005 edition was eliminated. Since the last edition there has not been conclusive evidence to prove the validity of the oral-motor approach in helping with the production of speech sounds.

Using *The SLP's IEP Companion*

The SLP's IEP Companion has 11 units that provide goals and objectives for many of the areas of speech–language pathology. Each unit begins with a rationale for the teaching of that topic and a description of the contents of the unit.

Most units are divided into sections containing subtopics. Each section begins with a yearly goal followed by objectives and a specific example of how to teach each objective. Some of the yearly goals are broken into short-term goals. These too are followed by objectives and examples.

The sections, goals, and objectives are in developmental order. Each section begins with goals and objectives for the youngest child who may need intervention in that area and proceeds to higher developmental levels for older students. Pragmatics is the first unit because it is the most general area of language.

Selecting Objectives

Following an assessment of an individual's communication abilities, establish appropriate goals and objectives by choosing appropriate units and sections from *The SLP's IEP Companion* as a guide. The guide is helpful whether planning an IEP for a public school student or an intervention program for a patient or client in another setting. Choose as many objectives as needed to construct a balanced plan for individualized intervention.

For example, when you are planning for a first-grade student diagnosed with delay in syntactic-morphological development and phonological awareness deficits that interfere with reading progress in her first-grade classroom, it could be appropriate to select goals from three sections: Phonological Awareness, Past Tense Verbs, and Narrative Discourse Skills in Children and Adolescents. As objectives are achieved, add additional objectives to the student's plan until dismissal is recommended. In this way, it is possible to write a sequential plan in a format that will become a record of the student's communication growth.

Using the Intervention Objectives

Individual objectives follow yearly goals. The objectives are designed to help the student achieve the yearly goal. Examples of practical intervention follow each objective in order to show (one example of) how the individual objective could be achieved. Intervention objectives assist the professional to work as a team alongside parents and other educators to reach communication goals. Team planning and instruction lead to multiple opportunities for students to achieve language competence. For students in a school setting, speech and language seems more important when integrated into the curriculum of the school day.

Writing Measureable Objectives

The language of the objectives in *The SLP's IEP Companion* is the basis for the performance objectives you will write for individual students. Use the objectives in *The SLP's IEP Companion* as guides to create personalized therapy plans for your students. When writing behavioral objectives to create an individualized objective, specify the following information:

- Name of the individual (Who will achieve the objective?)
- Specific task to be accomplished (What will this student achieve?)
- Specific result expected (What percentage will the student achieve?)
- Conditions (Who will assist in achieving the objectives?)
- Media and materials needed (What materials will be used to help the student achieve criteria?)
- Measurement of success (What instruments will be used to assess progress?)

Here is an example of a measurable objective:

> When presented with 10 picture pairs of objects from the same category, Greg will say the name of a category to tell how the two objects are similar with 80% accuracy during three consecutive lessons as assessed by the SLP or classroom teacher.

The SLP's IEP Companion is a valuable tool to help professionals from many backgrounds work together to improve communication abilities in children, adolescents, and adults. This reference can be used not only as a guide for creating individualized plans but also for structuring lessons in a hierarchical sequence. Its objectives contain hundreds of ideas that can be adapted to specific situations. The appendixes include practical lists and tools. Whatever communication difficulties your students, patients, or clients have, it is our hope that this resource will save you valuable professional time and give you a basis for collaborative educational planning.

Carolyn and Janet

Unit 1

Pragmatics

- Nonverbal Communication in Nonverbal Children
- Beginning Communicative Intentions: One-Word Stage
- Conversational Acts in Preschool Children
- Conversational Acts in School-Age Children and Adolescents
- Nonverbal Communication in Verbal Children and Adolescents
- Social Interaction Skills
- Classroom Communication Skills
- Classroom Social Survival Skills
- Narrative Discourse

Watching language unfold in children is a wonder to observe. At only 2 months of age, a baby begins babbled sounds that soon lead to conversational babbling and cooing. The baby quickly learns the pattern of speaking–listening–speaking with another person, and *pragmatics* is born. Children soon learn that they can communicate—that there are reasons to talk, things to talk about, and people to talk with. We are using pragmatics (Owens, 2016, p. 22) when we use language to affect others or relay information to them. How early it begins!

Children who live in an environment rich in loving connections with others use all that is available to them to reach out and connect with other people and affect their behavior. They use gestures, movements, facial expressions, sounds, and, finally, recognizable words. Later, their developing semantics and syntax become a part of their repertoire to connect their ideas as a way to influence others.

Pragmatics is the most general area of language because the purpose of language is to affect others, whether through pictures, words, signs, gestures, posture, facial expressions, or writing. Listening, sound production, syntax and morphology, vocabulary and semantics, and social skills all exist to give us a means to connect with others—to communicate. Speakers who know how to use language appropriately have gone past linguistic competence, however. They have *communicative competence* (Gleason & Ratner, 2013, p. 18).

When children do not develop language through interacting with others and exploring their environment, they need the help of many professionals. They "often have difficulty regulating and expressing their own emotions" (Power-deFur, 2016, p. 58). Parents and caregivers may need direction for early enrichment experiences with their children. Gestures, pictures, and signs may need to be taught to enhance abilities to interact until speaking is possible. Individualized treatment plans are needed to help these children communicate. The pragmatic success of an utterance has to do with its communicative effectiveness and appropriateness. Both aspects, effectiveness and appropriateness, are often reduced in children who have language disorders. These deficits may be related to gaps in any of the developing areas of communication mentioned earlier.

In planning pragmatics intervention, professionals may find it helpful to think of a child's communication problems with pragmatics on two continua: conversational assertiveness and conversational responsiveness. Conversational *assertiveness* is the ability or willingness to take a conversational turn, even when a child's conversational partner doesn't initiate it. Conversational *responsiveness* is the ability or willingness to meet the needs of a conversational partner by responding verbally to the partner's request for action or simply acknowledging a partner's comment. Observation of the child's tendencies toward assertiveness or responsiveness can help intervention planning.

See Figure 1.1, "Different Patterns of Social-Conversational Activity," adapted from the work of Fey (1986). The figure depicts the social-conversational continua of assertiveness and responsiveness. Assertiveness and responsiveness have to do with initiating, maintaining, and extending a topic. *Assertiveness* is the ability or willingness to take a conversational turn when none has been solicited by a partner. It includes both requestives (asking for information clarification, action, or attention) and assertives (commenting, explaining, giving rules, telling own thoughts, disagreeing, etc.). *Responsiveness* is the ability or willingness to respond to the needs of the conversational partner. It includes responsives (attempting to give information requested by the partner, responding verbally to the request for the action by the partner whether taking action or not, or simply acknowledging a comment by the partner). Responsives are in some way contingent on a prior request.

Active Conversationalists	**Passive Conversationalists**
+ Conversational Assertiveness + Conversational Responsiveness The child is generally both appropriately assertive and responsive during conversations. + Frequent assertive conversational acts. High rate of asking for information, actions, clarification, or attention. High rate of giving facts, information, etc. Frequent topic initiations. + High rates of responding to the partner's assertives or requestives. Much willingness to attend to the details of the partner's requests and comments and to consider those details in formulating responses in order to maintain or extend a conversation.	– Conversational Assertiveness + Conversational Responsiveness The child is responsive but nonassertive during conversations. – Low rates of asking for information, actions, clarification, or attention. Low rate of giving facts, information, etc. Low rate of topic initiations. + High rates of responding to the partner's assertives or requestives. Much willingness to attend to the details of the partner's requests and comments and to consider those details in formulating responses in order to maintain or extend a conversation.
Verbal Noncommunicators	**Inactive Communicators**
+ Conversational Assertiveness – Conversational Responsiveness The child is generally assertive but nonresponsive during conversations. + Frequent assertive conversational acts. High rate of asking for information, actions, clarification, or attention. High rate of giving facts, information, etc. Frequent topic initiations. – Low rates of attending to the partner's assertions. Low rate of willingness to attend to the details of the partner's responsives and to consider those details in formulating responses to maintain or extend the conversation. – High tendency to initiate new topics or attempt to maintain or extend topics with information that is minimally related to the partner's prior request or comment.	– Conversational Assertiveness – Conversational Responsiveness The child is neither assertive nor responsive during conversations. – Low rates of asking for information, actions, clarification, or attention. Low rate of giving facts, information, etc. Low rate of topic initiations. – Low rates of responding to the partner's assertives and requestives. Little willingness to attend to the partner's requests and comments. Few attempts to maintain or extend the conversation by considering those details in formulating or making responses.

Figure 1.1. Different patterns of social-conversational activity. Adapted from *Language Intervention With Young Children*, by M. Fey, 1986, San Diego, CA: College-Hill Press.

Each quadrant in Figure 1.1 represents a group of children whose social-conversational activity shows a distinct pattern. By applying clinical observation and test results of the student's conversational participation, professionals can use the chart to help determine basic pragmatic intervention objectives. Intervention can then be designed to increase responsiveness or meaningful assertiveness in conversation.

This unit provides a framework of objectives designed for use by speech–language pathologists (SLPs) and language specialists who plan intervention in pragmatics. The scope of the objectives is broad. It spans pragmatic behaviors in nonverbal children (e.g., gestures, body postures, facial expressions), beginning intentional language at the one-word level, speech acts in young children, conversational acts in children and adolescents, nonverbal communication in verbal children, social interaction skills, classroom communication skills, classroom social behavior, and narrative discourse skills.

Children's stories and pictures are filled with examples of social interactions that you can use to support intervention for pragmatics by talking about the stories or using them for role play. Using visual organizers with stories can support your work with social interaction. This is especially true when characters in the stories must solve problems through communication. See Appendix C for concept maps used as visual organizers.

Description of Contents

Nonverbal Communication in Nonverbal Children. The objectives in this section are for use with preverbal or nonverbal individuals who can use gestures, pictures, and vocalizations to communicate intentions. The system chosen for use in these objectives is from Miller (1981), an adaptation of Coggins and Carpenter (1981), who defined eight pragmatic categories identifiable in preverbal or nonverbal children.

Beginning Communicative Intentions: One-Word Stage. This section's objectives are for children whose developmental stage allows them to use communication behaviors and single words to communicate their intentions.

Conversational Acts in Preschool Children. These objectives are for children whose developmental stage allows them to use communication behaviors and sentences to function as a speaker and a listener in interactions. Children at this stage choose what to say and how to say it, suit their language to the social environment, have many reasons for speaking, and speak in relationship to another to add to the conversation.

Conversational Acts in School-Age Children and Adolescents. Objectives in this section are designed for children whose developmental stage allows them to use conversational rules. Becoming a competent conversationalist requires a complex set of skills. Children must learn, for example, that a competent listener has an active role in maintaining conversation. They learn rules, among others, for turn taking, topic maintenance, asking for and giving clarification, avoiding interrupting, and using a casual style versus a formal style.

Nonverbal Communication in Verbal Children and Adolescents. Use these objectives to help children develop the ability to understand and use nonverbal means to express desires, needs, and emotions: postures, gestures; facial expressions; space, touch; time; rhythm; and vocal tone, intensity, and loudness. They are for students who are able to understand that messages can be conveyed nonverbally.

Social Interaction Skills. These objectives are designed for children whose developmental stage allows them to use language to deal with more complex relationships. These social skills are important as children and adolescents learn to become effective members of their culture. The ability to develop interactive skills allows children access to social interaction with peers and makes a positive impression with teachers and other powerful adults.

Classroom Communication Skills. This section's objectives are for students who are able to interact with peers and teachers in the school environment. Like adults, children have to learn the rules of specific conversational genres. Classroom discourse skills are demanded of children if they are to be successful at school.

This section includes objectives specific to classroom discourse: listening, speaking, asking and answering questions, and so on.

Classroom Social Survival Skills. These objectives continue the previous objectives for classroom communication skills. These objectives are more specific, however, to fulfilling teacher expectations that students will participate in the classroom routine (e.g., stay on task, be responsible) and relate effectively to the teacher (e.g., use active listening, work quietly, ask for help).

Narrative Discourse. See objectives in this section for children of all ages who can listen to and develop even the most basic storytelling skills. *Narrative discourse* is the ability to translate knowing what has happened into telling about it (Naremore, Densmore, & Harman, 2001). Children use narratives when they report what has happened as they create "stories" that can be either factual or imaginary (Appel & Masterson, 1998). Narrative discourse skills support reading and writing skills. Strong (1998) reported that young students who have practice in understanding and telling stories move more easily from oral language to literacy skills in school. Part 1 objectives are for younger children, preschool–Grade 3, that range from developing simple scripts for familiar events to retelling stories with several episodes. Part 2 objectives are for older students, Grades 3–8. The objectives include telling and writing original stories using all elements of basic story grammar and cohesion, as shown in Appendix C.

Nonverbal Communication in Nonverbal Children

Yearly Goal: *To use intentional nonverbal means (gestures, vocalizations, and pictures) to communicate with a listener*

Note: These objectives are appropriate for preverbal or nonverbal individuals of all ages who can use gestures, pictures, or vocalizations to communicate intentions.

Objectives	Examples
1. Watches speaker's face when spoken to.	SLP: **Hi, Nathan. Look at me. Look here.** S: Looks at the speaker's face.
2. Uses gestures or vocalizations to gain attention.	SLP: Ignores the child while playing with something the child might want. S: Gestures or vocalizes to get the SLP's attention.
3. Directs a listener to provide some object by using gestures, vocalizations, or pictures.	SLP: **Show me what you want.** S: Reaches for, points to, or uses eye gaze or a picture to request an object or food.
4. Directs a listener to make an object move by using gestures, vocalizations, or pictures. (The action, not the object, is the student's focus of interest.)	SLP: **Watch my windup toy. What should we do now?** S: Gestures to get the SLP to make the toy move again.
5. Imitates actions.	SLP: Claps hands or stomps feet to the beat of the music. S: Imitates the actions.
6. Greets and expresses recognition or indicates goodbye by using gestures, vocalizations, or pictures when a person enters a room.	SLP: **Hi, Gregory!** S: Gestures and uses facial expressions for a greeting.
7. Expresses an intention to give someone else an object by using gestures, vocalizations, or pictures.	SLP: **Let's share this toy. I'm going to share it with Ellie. Now you show me how you give it to Ellie.** S: Holds the toy out toward Ellie to indicate a desire to give it to her.
8. Shows frustration when not understood.	SLP: **Let's pretend it is snack time. You are saying what you want to drink, but the snack leader does not understand you. Show me how it makes you feel.** S: Points to a picture of someone who is mad. SLP: **Here are some things you can do. Point to the drink again. Hand the snack leader a picture of the drink you want.**
9. Acknowledges the listener's previous comments were received by using gestures, vocalizations, or pictures.	SLP: **Parker, when Natalie says something to you, do this so she will know that you heard her:** SLP: Makes eye contact and nods head. S: Nods, vocalizes, or uses other nonverbal means to indicate that he heard what was said.

(continues)

Objectives	Examples
10. Responds to a request for information from the listener by using gestures, vocalizations, or pictures.	SLP: **It's time for a snack. Who wants juice?** S: Responds by using positive or negative gestures, vocalizations, or pictures.
11. Directs a listener to provide information about an object, action, or location by using gestures, vocalizations, or pictures.	SLP: Covers part of a page with her hand or paper. S: Pushes the obstruction away and vocalizes to ask for more information.

Beginning Communicative Intentions: One-Word Stage

Yearly Goal: *To use intentional social communication behaviors and words to communicate intentions interactively with a listener*

Objectives	Examples
1. Labels objects, events, and locations while indicating each one to a listener.	S: While playing with toys, shows a doll to the listener and says **baby**.
2. Answers a speaker's question by labeling an object or person, showing by eye gaze and gestures that the word is in response to the question.	SLP: While playing with toys: **What's that?** S: Holds the toy up and says **choo-choo**.
3. Requests that a listener perform an action, using a word and gestures to indicate the desired action.	SLP: Playing with a toy car: **What do you want the car to do?** S: **Go!**
4. Requests an answer from the listener using a word and gestures to indicate an answer is expected.	SLP: Hides the ball they are playing with. S: Searches and says **Ball?** with rising intonation to indicate **Where is the ball?**
5. Calls a person's name to get that person's attention.	SLP: As S plays with toys. Dad is in the room: **Do you want Daddy to come over and play with you? Look at him like this and say "Daddy."** S: Looks at him and says **Daddy**.
6. Greets a person with eye contact, facial expressions, and a word, such as the person's name or "Hi."	SLP: **Here comes Mommy. Remember to look at her and say "Hi."** S: Moves toward mother and says **Hi**.
7. Uses a protest word, gestures, or postures to express displeasure, desire for an action to stop, or refusal of an object or action (shakes head, pushes object away, or uses another negative gesture and says "No!").	SLP: Offers S a cracker. **If you don't want the cracker, shake your head like this and say "No."** S: Pushes the cracker away, shakes head, and says **No**.
8. Refers to self by name.	SLP: Pointing to a picture of the child: **Who is this?** S: **Anna**
9. Calls attention to self or own actions ("Mommy! See!").	SLP: **If you want me to look at your blocks, point to them and say "See!"** S: Points to stacked blocks and says **See!**

Objectives	Examples
10. Exhibits verbal turn taking.	SLP: Rolls ball to child and says **ball**. S: Rolls ball back to SLP and makes a vocalization such as **ba** or **ball**. This sequence is repeated over and over also using other words, such as *roll* or *go*.
11. During play, talks to self, imitates adult play behaviors, and engages in simple pretend play.	SLP: Picks up a toy phone, says **Hi**, pretends to talk, and hands the phone to the child. S: Imitates the SLP's actions and also pretends to talk on the phone.
12. Practices intonation, sometimes imitating an adult.	SLP: **It's snack time. Do you want a cookie? Say it like this: "cookie?"** (with rising intonation to indicate *May I have a cookie?*). S: Says **cookie?** with rising intonation.

Conversational Acts in Preschool Children

Yearly Goal: *To participate as a listener or speaker in a variety of meaningful conversational acts—responses and assertions—using syntax and articulation at the child's developmental level*

Objectives	Examples
Short-Term Goal: Makes meaningful responses as the listener in interactions with a speaker using developmentally appropriate loudness, intonation, facial expressions, and gestures	
1. Responds to a request for attention.	SLP: **It's circle time, Adam.** S: Responds nonverbally or verbally by looking up, joining the circle, or saying *yes* or *what*.
2. Responds to a request for his name with appropriate eye contact and by saying his name.	SLP: **Let's practice what you will say when the new librarian asks your name. She will say "What's your name?" and you will say "Julian."** S: In response to being asked his name, says **Julian**.
3. Responds to a request for his age with appropriate eye contact and by saying his age.	SLP: **If someone asks "How old are you?" you can hold up four fingers or say "four." Let's practice. How old are you, Oliver?** S: Looks at the speaker and says **four**.
4. Responds to a request for an action with an appropriate verbal and/or nonverbal response.	SLP: **We will play a following-directions game: Listen and do what I say. Jamie, jump three times.** S: Says **okay** and jumps three times.
5. Responds to a compliment by saying "thank you."	SLP: **It's circle time. Let's go around the circle, and I will give each of you a compliment. Sophia, I like your hair today.** S: Looks at SLP and says **thank you**.

(continues)

Objectives	Examples
6. Responds to acknowledge information given by the speaker.	SLP: **It's Shirley's turn for show-and-tell.** S: Listens to Shirley, looks at her, and makes a comment about her show-and-tell item.
7. Responds verbally and nonverbally to indirect requests in a variety of settings and situations.	SLP: **When I say something, you can reply to me. For example, I might say "I'm hungry" and you could say "Let's have a snack." Let's try one. I'm cold.** S: Gets a sweater and says **Here is your sweater.**
Short-Term Goal: Makes meaningful requests and comments as a speaker in an interaction using developmentally appropriate loudness, intonation, facial expressions, and gestures	
8. Greets others or says "bye" appropriately in a variety of settings and situations.	SLP: **Let's take a walk around school. When we see someone on our walk, you should look at them and tell them "Hi."** S: **Hi, Mr. Baird.**
9. Calls for a listener's attention before speaking.	SLP: **Out on the playground when you want someone to play with you, say his name first.** S: **Hey, Justin. Let's play!**
10. Requests an object of the listener.	SLP: **We will practice how to ask for things. If you want something from your teacher, say her name first.** S: **Mrs. Tade, may I have the blue crayon?**
11. Requests an action of the listener.	SLP: **When you are in the library, remember to say Mrs. Bryant's name first.** S: **Mrs. Bryant, will you help me find a dog book?**
12. Requests the speaker to clarify a comment.	SLP: **I'm going to say something that you cannot hear well or understand. Should you say "What" or "Huh"?** S: **No.** SLP: **You can say "What did you say?" "Could you say that again?" or "I don't understand."**
13. Gives compliments appropriately.	SLP: **It is circle time. Look at the person next to you and give him or her a compliment. I will start. David, I like your new shoes!** S: **Scott, the picture you drew is really good!**
14. Uses indirect speech acts to soften speech.	SLP: **We will practice polite speech. I'm going to say some things nicely and some things that don't sound nice. Hold up a happy face or sad face to show which one you think it is: "Get me some milk." "I think we need some milk." Then you will say some and I will hold up the faces.** S: Holds up sad face then happy face and then says **May I borrow your book? Hey, I want that book.**

Objectives	Examples
15. Denies a statement made by someone else or indicates noncompliance with a request.	SLP: **I'm going to say some things during our game that are not true, and we will practice what you should say: It's my turn.** S: **No, it's my turn.**
Short-Term Goal: Makes statements to label, give facts, explain feelings, and make explanations	
16. Labels familiar objects at the appropriate vocabulary level.	SLP: **Look around the playground. Tell me some things that you see.** S: **I see swings. That's a tall slide.**
17. Labels actions at the appropriate vocabulary level.	SLP: **Everyone is working on a different craft. Tell me what you and the other children are doing.** S: **I color. Brady is cutting paper.**
18. Comments about events.	SLP: **It's time to put the toys away. Tell me about what you are doing.** S: **The ball goes here. I put up the markers.**
19. Describes present events.	SLP: **What is happening in this barnyard picture?** S: **The cow is mooing. The farmer is digging.**
20. Describes a past event.	SLP: **Take turns around the circle and tell what we did on our field trip to the zoo.** S: **We rode on a bus. We saw some tigers.**
21. Teases, jokes, warns, claims, exclaims, or conveys humor ("You can't catch me! Watch out! It's my turn now").	SLP: **Let's say some funny things about the jungle animal video. What if the giraffe barked?** S: **What if the zebra gave the elephant his stripes?**
22. Uses imagination or fantasy in play after hearing a story or taking part in an event.	SLP: **Let's act out the Goldilocks story we just read. You are Mama Bear, Don is Baby Bear, Matthew is Papa Bear, and Vanessa is Goldilocks.** S: The children act out the story, using special voices for their characters.

Conversational Acts in School-Age Children and Adolescents

Yearly Goal: *To participate effectively in conversations with peers and adults so that their own intentions are communicated and intentions of others are correctly interpreted*

CCSS.ELA-LITERACY.SL.K.2–SL.1.2
CCSS.ELA-LITERACY.SL.2.3
CCSS.ELA-LITERACY.SL.3.1.C

Objectives	Examples
Short-Term Goal: Uses rituals of the culture for beginning and ending conversations	
1. Uses formal or casual language to suit conversational partners and situations.	SLP: **There will be some people coming by to visit our class tomorrow. When they come, is it okay to welcome them like we do our friends? Go line up outside the door and we will pretend you are the visitors. Tell me if the way I greet you is good or not: (1) Hey there! (2) Hello, Mr. Brown. We are glad you are here.** S: Decides if the greetings are appropriate or not and practices some good ones.
2. Uses a tone of voice appropriate to the situation.	SLP: **We are going to practice changing our tone of voice to make the same words mean different things. You are going to say "That's a great idea." The card you choose will tell you what tone of voice to use:** S: Practices saying the phrase with these tones of voice: excited, sarcastic, friendly, bragging, sad, disappointed.
3. Greets others and says farewells in a friendly way.	SLP: **Let's use these puppets to practice telling friends hello and goodbye. Remember to have them look at each other and smile.** S: Using puppets: **Hi. What's up? How are you today? So long. See you later.**
4. Attends to a speaker with appropriate eye contact, gestures, and responses that indicate good listening.	SLP: **Let's list some ways you can show the speaker that you are a good listener in a conversation.** S: **Use good eye contact, nod, have a listening body posture, and make comments.**
5. Introduces self to others.	SLP: **A new student will join our class tomorrow. What is a good way to let her know your name?** S: **Go up to the new student and say, "Welcome to our class. I'm Jon."**
6. Introduces others and invites them to join in conversations.	SLP: **Mark, how would you include Tucker in a group of your other friends who don't know him?** S: **This is my friend, Tucker. He just moved here from Santa Fe.**

Objectives	Examples
7. Joins in conversations started by others.	SLP: **Have you ever walked up to a group of people and wanted to join in the conversation? You first need to listen to what they are talking about and then add a comment. Pretend that a group is talking about a new movie. What could you say?** S: **I liked that movie, too.**
8. Initiates conversations by getting the person's attention and choosing an appropriate topic.	SLP: **If you want to start a conversation with someone, you should walk over to him, look at him, say "hi," and talk about something that is interesting to both of you. Practice by starting a conversation with me.** S: Gets SLP's attention with eye contact and says, **Hi. Are you coming to the school open house tonight?**
9. Invites others into conversations.	SLP: **Let's pretend that you are talking to Rachel. Andrea walks up and wants to join the conversation you are having about a movie. How could you help her?** S: **Andrea, Rachel, and I are talking about the movie we saw last night. Have you seen any good movies lately?**
10. Leaves conversations in a friendly way.	SLP: **If you are having a conversation with someone and want to leave it, it is not polite to just walk away. You should tell why you are ending the conversation and suggest you can talk again later. Pretend you are talking with a friend on the telephone. What could you say to end it?** S: **I need to finish my homework. Let's talk tomorrow at school. Bye.**
11. Plans, initiates, and responds to telephone calls.	SLP: **Telephone skills are special because you cannot see one another. When you call someone on the phone, you need to identify yourself, use the person's name, and begin and end the conversation in a friendly way. Try one.** S: **Hi, Jody. This is Jeff. Can you talk now? Catch you later. Bye.**
Short-Term Goal: Participates in and maintains a conversation topic	
12. Stays on topic and avoids changing the topic abruptly.	SLP: **Staying on topic helps everyone enjoy a conversation. Let's talk about our visit to the wildlife center. I'll begin: It surprised me to see so many antelopes running across the wildlife prairie.** S1: **I laughed when the giraffes came right up to the tour truck.** S2: **The fawns were so tiny and cute.**

(continues)

Objectives	Examples
13. Changes a topic appropriately.	SLP: **After staying on topic for a while, it's okay to change the topic in a friendly way. Go ahead and change the topic from the wildlife center.** S: **Last night I saw a movie about lions. Really funny! What did you do last night, Aaron?**
14. Avoids interrupting others and ignores inappropriate interruptions of others.	SLP: **There is a polite way to handle interruptions in a conversation. Let's practice. Veronica and Sarah, pretend you're talking after school. I'll interrupt you. How could you resist being interrupted in a friendly way?** S: **I could say, "Hi, Ms. SLP. Just a moment, Nora has to leave." I could say, "Bye, Nora," and then tell you hello.**
15. Takes turns being a speaker and listener.	SLP: **Today we'll play the Ball of String game to practice taking turns speaking and listening. While you hold the ball, you speak; others listen. Then toss it to someone else, and it's his or her turn to talk.** Sam: **Hi, Mark. What did you do this weekend?** Mark: **I went fishing. Do you fish, Rachel?** Rachel: **Yes, I've caught fish at City Lake.**
Short-Term Goal: Knows and uses four conversational maxims: Be concise, honest, relevant, and clear	
16. Gives just enough information and avoids dominating a conversation.	SLP: **There are maxims to help us learn about having a conversation. Here's the first one: Be concise. That means to give enough details but don't do all the talking. Let's talk about our trip to the park and practice being concise. Logan, you begin.** S: **I thought the best part of the field trip was eating lunch at the park. Something funny happened to Rachel. Tell them, Rachel!**
17. Judges own amount of information and determines by listener's responses if it is too little or too much.	SLP: **You can find out if you gave the right amount of information by watching your listener's actions and facial expressions. How can you tell?** S: **I could ask myself, is my listener smiling and looking interested? I'll continue. Is he yawning or looking away? I'll stop.**
18. Gives truthful information and avoids superimposing own views and opinions as though factual ("I'll be honest").	SLP: **Here is the second maxim: Be honest. Don't give your *views* as *facts*. How could you let your listeners know the difference?** S: **I could say, "This is my opinion, but I think chocolate ice cream is the best dessert flavor!"**

Objectives	Examples
19. Makes relevant remarks and avoids superimposing own obsessive interests on a conversation ("I'll be relevant").	SLP: **"Be relevant" is the third maxim. This means that it's important to add to a topic under discussion, not direct it. Perhaps you love to talk about science fiction, but the topic is about space travel. How can you resist changing the topic to science fiction?** S: **I could tell myself, I love to talk about science fiction, but the topic is space travel. I'll stay on the group's topic, space travel.**
20. Judges own clarity and listener's responses to determine if the listener is understanding ("I'll be clear").	SLP: **"Be clear" is the fourth maxim. It's important to ask yourself, does my listener understand me? Can you tell about a time when you needed to make yourself clear?** S: **I said to Rosita, "I saw it every night when we were in the desert." She looked confused. So I said, "I saw the space station every night."**
Short-Term Goal: Repairs communication breakdowns	
21. Asks for and gives more information when needed.	SLP: **Sometimes you may need to ask friends questions when you don't understand a message. You need to ask for clarification. Now ask me for more information.** S: **What does *clarification* mean?** SLP: **Good question. It means to make the message easier to understand by telling more about it.**
22. Politely asks the speaker to repeat when needed, such as when information was not heard.	SLP: **Sometimes we may not hear clearly what a speaker has said. If so, we should ask in a friendly way for the speaker to repeat. Suppose you didn't hear a new friend's name. In a friendly way, show me what you would say.** S: **I'm sorry, I didn't catch your name.**
23. Knows when to ask for clarification when he or she does not understand the speaker.	SLP: **During a conversation we may become confused about what someone said. How do you know when to ask for clarification?** S: **When I don't understand what she means.**
24. Politely asks for clarification when needed.	SLP: **On our next test you will compare characters from the book. Does everyone understand?** S: **I'm sorry, but I didn't get the date of the test.**

Nonverbal Communication in Verbal Children and Adolescents

Yearly Goal: *To understand and use nonverbal communication to express desires, needs, and emotions*

Note: These objectives are appropriate for verbal individuals at many different ability levels.

Objectives	Examples
Short-Term Goal: Understands and uses effective paralanguage (pitch, stress, rate, intensity)	
1. Interprets the differences in meaning conveyed by tone of voice, intensity, rate, and pitch.	SLP: **Choose one of the cards from my stack and then say this sentence with tone of voice, intensity, rate, and pitch that show the meaning on the card. The sentence is "I came in second place."** S: Says the sentence conveying one of these meanings: joy, sadness, surprise, disappointment, or fear, and the other students guess the meaning.
2. Analyzes use of pitch, stress, rate, and intensity.	SLP: **While we plan our play of *Goldilocks and the Three Bears*, let's talk about how each character would use pitch, stress, rate, and intensity.** S: **Father Bear would use a loud, slow, low-pitched voice to show us that he is big and confident and in charge.**
Short-Term Goal: Understands and uses facial expressions appropriately	
3. Understands and demonstrates the difference between appropriate eye contact and staring.	SLP: **Today we will take turns staring and also using appropriate eye contact while having a conversation. What effect did each kind of eye contact have on our conversation?** S: **Appropriate eye contact: This showed interest in the conversation. Staring: This made me uncomfortable and made it more difficult to pay attention to the conversation.**
4. Determines the attitudes that are conveyed by demonstrations of emotions through facial expressions, such as serious, relaxed, or disturbed.	SLP: **Let's sit in a circle. We will take turns using different facial expressions to show different emotions. The rest of us will guess the emotion.** S: Takes turns showing facial expressions that convey happy, sad, serious, sleepy, scared, and so on.

Objectives	Examples
Short-Term Goal: Understands and uses space appropriately	
5. Understands and uses personal space to avoid invading others' personal space and to protect his or her own space.	SLP: **The space around your body is called *your personal space*. If you get too close to someone or he or she gets too close to you, it's called *invasion of personal space*. It can make you feel uncomfortable. Let's practice standing and talking to each other. Show your partner how close is comfortable for you.** S: Stands too close to and then a comfortable distance from a conversation partner and tells how it feels.
6. Comprehends and appropriately uses space in four spatial zones: intimate (within 18 inches), personal (18 inches–4 feet), social (4 feet–12 feet), and public (beyond 12 feet).	SLP: **These lines taped on the floor show appropriate distances to stand from other people. With a partner, we are going to demonstrate the proper and improper use of the personal zone in everyday settings. Tell what situations would be good for each distance.** S: Stands with a partner at each distance. **Within 18 inches: Family and close friends.** **18 inches to 4 feet: Talking to a teacher about homework.** **4 feet to 12 feet: Talking to a friend on the playground.** **12 feet and beyond: Getting the attention of someone in the distance by using gestures and postures until the person gets closer.**
Short-Term Goal: Understands and uses touch appropriately	
7. Understands and uses societal rules regarding touch.	SLP: **The way we touch one another has different meanings. I will act out a kind of touch, and you can tell me what it means.** S: Tells what these kinds of touch mean: a pat on the back (encouragement), shaking someone (anger), kicking (anger), a handshake (friendliness), and so on.
8. Develops awareness that everyone has a right to determine who touches him or her and that one's body and personal space must be respected.	SLP: **It's important for you to know that you get to decide who can and can't touch you. Let's list some.** S: **Can: Parents, close friends, adults you trust.** **Can't: Strangers, someone you don't trust.**

(continues)

Objectives	Examples
Short-Term Goal: Understands and effectively uses body language (posture and gesture)	
9. Interprets and uses postures (body orientation) and gestures (use of head, arms, fingers, legs, and shoulders) to send nonverbal messages.	SLP: **With your partner use body language such as gestures and postures to signal the meaning of these messages: stop, come here, quiet down, comfort me, don't come near me, and I have confidence.** S: Uses gestures and postures that indicate each message.
10. Discusses and defines emotions and how they are conveyed nonverbally: anger, sadness, seriousness, disgust, fear, happiness, relief, and disappointment.	SLP: **We'll look at body language in these cartoon characters. Before you read the words in the cartoon, decide the feeling of the character in each frame.** S: **This character with a happy face is motioning to a puppy. He is happy and wants the puppy to come to him.**
11. Understands and uses posture and gestures to send nonverbal messages.	SLP: **Look at yourself in this full-length mirror. Send a nonverbal message by standing with your hands on your hips. What message are you sending?** S: **My mind is made up. I mean what I say!**
Short-Term Goal: Understands and effectively uses body rhythm and speech rate.	
12. Understands that certain situations require a slow rate of speech and others require a fast rate of speech.	SLP: **Our speech rate sends messages. Tell me which speech rate is appropriate for each situation:** **1. Walking in the school hallway** **2. Responding to a fire drill** **3. Walking with a large group of people in the shopping mall** S: **(1) slow, (2) fast, (3) slow.**
13. Mimics varying rhythms in speaking and walking.	SLP: **We watched a movie scene where characters had various rates of speaking and walking. Imitate the speaking rate and rhythm for the villain and the good guy.** S: Imitates the villain's fast rate and jerky rhythm, then the good guy's slow, confident rate and rhythm.

Objectives	Examples
Short-Term Goal: Understands and uses time appropriately	
14. Understands that the use of time is one way we communicate to others and that people often have a negative perception of those who are not able to judge time and use it properly.	SLP: **The way we use time gives positive and negative messages that we might not intend to make. Tell whether these messages are positive or negative:** **1. A person is 10 minutes late to class.** **2. A person comes to a party 30 minutes early.** **3. A student turns in a report on the day it is due.** S: **(1) negative, (2) negative, (3) positive.**
15. Distinguishes time-related situations when the pace picks up or slows down.	SLP: **The amount of time we have affects how fast we talk. Would speech rate pick up or slow down in each situation?** **1. Your bus leaves in 5 minutes.** **2. Your mom calls to tell you she will be 20 minutes late picking you up.** **3. A fire alarm sounded.** S: **(1) pick up, (2) slow down, (3) pick up.**

Social Interaction Skills

Yearly Goal: *To use social interaction skills to communicate and respond to the feelings, intents, and needs of self and others in order to interpret and communicate feelings, use self-control, and deal with stress*

Objectives	Examples
Short-Term Goal: Deals with feelings in ways that meet the needs of self and others	
1. Recognizes a variety of personal positive feelings, such as happy, hopeful, eager, sympathetic, excited, generous, kind, and brave, and negative feelings, such as angry, irritated, afraid, alarmed, tearful, sad, lonely, and fearful.	SLP: **Think about the many ways your body feels during a day. Does your body get tight when you feel anxious? How does your body let you know you are afraid? You're happy?** S: **When I'm afraid my hands get sweaty. When I'm happy I feel light and my face smiles easily.**
2. Uses feeling words to describe personal feelings.	SLP: **Think about your day. Name the feelings you've had so far today and tell the reasons.** S: **Today I felt relieved when I passed the test and embarrassed when I fell down the steps. I was excited when Dad said, "You may go out with your friends."**

(continues)

Objectives	Examples
3. Recognizes and labels feelings and moods of others by making inferences about a person's nonverbal cues.	SLP: **Did you like the class play? How did Nina probably feel at the beginning of the play? How could you tell?** S: **She felt excited and happy. She jumped up and down and squealed when her brother gave her a puppy for her birthday.**
4. Controls anger with peers and adults.	SLP: **Controlling anger can be tricky. Think about the feelings in our story. Samuel's little brother spilled milk on his sandwich. Samuel yelled at his little brother and made him cry. How else could Samuel have handled his anger?** S: **He could have waited to say anything until he felt calm.**
5. Handles fear constructively rather than becoming immobilized by it.	SLP: **Let's talk about facing our fear rather than avoiding what we fear, such as giving a speech. What good things could you tell yourself?** S: **My speech about bees will help my friends get ready for our test on bees. I have a good story to tell. I'll do just fine.**
6. Says positive things to self.	SLP: **Each of you has an important role to play when you're in a group. Write down ways you are contributing to your group.** S: (writes) I'm good at planning and sharing ideas. I listen to the others in the group.
7. Compliments another person.	SLP: **Do you like compliments? Most of us do. Suppose you want to tell José that you like his new shoes. How would you say it?** S: **Smile and say in a friendly way, "I like your new shoes!"**
8. Says "thank you" when complimented or praised.	SLP: **Suppose a friend likes your speech about bees. He says, "I learned some things about bees that I didn't know!" How could you sincerely receive the compliment?** S: **Simply say "thank you" in a friendly way.**
9. Offers to help others without taking over when help is both needed and wanted.	SLP: **How could you offer a friend help when you notice she is having a problem with a computer program?** S: **Say in a friendly way, "Would you like some help? I've used that program before."**

Objectives	Examples
10. Shares with others.	SLP: **Has someone ever shared kindly with you? Suppose you notice that a girl in your class forgot her umbrella, and she has to walk to the bus in the rain. What could you say?** S: **I noticed you don't have your umbrella. Would you like to share mine when we walk to the bus?**
11. Shows tolerance for persons with characteristics different from his or her own.	SLP: **We'll have a new student this week. He is from Haiti. How can we welcome him?** S: **We can smile and say "Hi." Play with him at recess. Sit with him at lunch. Be friendly.**
12. Deals with negative feelings of anger, fear, and disappointment.	SLP: **Disappointments can be tough. Let's suppose you're expecting your friend Sam to come over, but he doesn't come and doesn't even call. What could you do?** S: **I could stay away from self-put-downs. Tell myself, "I feel disappointed. I'll call him and see if he's okay."**
Short-Term Goal: Uses self-control and verbal methods as an alternative to aggression	
13. Takes the perspective of another person.	SLP: **Let's practice trying to see things through someone else's eyes. Suppose you're in a school study group. A friend sees a subject in a way completely different from the way you do. What could you say?** S: **I could say, "It makes sense how you could see it that way. Let's talk more."**
14. Asks permission before using belongings of others.	SLP: **Sometimes it may not feel necessary to ask permission to use others' equipment, but it's always necessary. Show us how you would ask permission to borrow a friend's marker.** S: **Matthew, may I borrow your red marker?**
15. Admits a mistake without shifting blame to others.	SLP: **Today we will practice admitting mistakes. Which sentence shows a responsible way to handle a mistake? (1) My parents forgot to sign my paper. (2) I forgot to get my paper signed.** S: **I forgot to get my paper signed.**
16. Accepts consequences for own mistakes and makes amends.	SLP: **Help Mark learn to accept consequences. He kept forgetting to return his overdue library book. The librarian refused to let him get another book. What should Mark do?** S: **Tell himself, "I feel bad about forgetting my book. I'll write myself a note so it won't happen again. I'll tell the librarian, 'I'm so sorry. I'll pay the fine.'"**

(continues)

Objectives	Examples
17. Handles false accusations appropriately.	SLP: **It's tough to be accused falsely. Let's talk about it. Suppose you returned your library book, but the librarian says it is not in the library. What could you do?** S: **I could tell her what happened. I returned the book, but I saw Anna Smith holding the same book on the bus this morning. It had a red ink mark on the cover just like the book I borrowed.**
18. Responds to teasing or name-calling by ignoring it, changing the subject, agreeing with the teaser, or using some other nonaggressive means.	SLP: **No one enjoys being teased. When you are teased by a peer, here's one thing you can do. Meet the teaser with quiet confidence. Agree with him. Let's practice. Suppose someone teases you by saying, "Your hair is so red! How could you stay cool?" What could you say?** S: **You're right. I have red hair.**
19. Responds to physical assault by leaving the situation, calling for help, or using some other constructive means.	SLP: **Danger can be real. We need to know that fear is often healthy. We can use fear wisely to get away or find help. It is never okay for someone to touch you or hurt you. If someone hits you or comes toward you with a weapon, what should you do?** S: **I should get away if I can and also yell for help. Then I need to get help from a teacher or another adult.**
20. Walks away from a peer when angry to avoid hitting.	SLP: **Sometimes we just need to walk away from conflict and cool off. Did that ever work for you? Write down some ways walking away can help you cool off and not lose control.** S: (writes) Walking away can help me keep from hitting someone. It gives me time to think about why I'm angry and find someone to talk to about the problem.
21. Expresses anger by telling the other person reasons for the anger, using nonaggressive words rather than physical action or aggressive words.	SLP: **How can we handle anger in healthy ways? Let's practice using polite words and a firm tone of voice even when we're angry. The goal is to get people to listen to you and change. Practice completing this sentence: I feel angry when _____ because _____.** S: **I would tell my brother, "I feel angry when you take my pencils without asking because then I have to search for a pencil to do my homework."**

Objectives	Examples
Short-Term Goal: Handles stressful situations with responsible actions	
22. Complies with directions of adults or peers in positions of authority.	SLP: **When teachers give directions, it's important for you to listen without complaining. What if you don't understand?** S: **Ask the teacher to clarify the directions. Then follow the directions without complaining.**
23. Accepts constructive criticism without giving up or lashing out.	SLP: **When a teacher suggests ways to improve your paper, why is it important to listen carefully and say "thank you"?** S: **The teacher wants to help me improve. It's courteous to tell her "thank you."**
24. Asks for help appropriately but only after trying to do an activity alone.	SLP: **Suppose you need help during class. You're reading an assignment in class when you discover a page has been ripped out of your book. Choose the correct answer: (1) I should blurt out, "Page 34 is ripped out of my book." (2) I should raise my hand and wait for the teacher.** S: **It's (2): Raise my hand and wait.**
25. Makes complaints confidently when things don't seem fair.	SLP: **Sometimes it's important to complain confidently. It was time for Ben to complain. During recess, students in Ben's class get to choose games, but Ethan always chooses volleyball. What could Ben say to the teacher to let her know what happens?** S: **He could go to the teacher privately and tell her "Ethan seems to get called on to choose most of the games. I'd like to choose, too."**
26. Apologizes and makes amends when own actions have hurt or infringed on another.	SLP: **Ethan didn't realize he was getting more turns to choose games than other students were. How could Ethan apologize and make amends for choosing all the games?** S: **He could say, "I'm sorry. I didn't realize I was choosing all the games. You take a turn."**
27. Takes action to deal with hurt feelings when left out by friends.	SLP: **Have you ever felt left out? It's easy to feel left out sometimes, even when a friend didn't intend to leave us out. Can you think of reasons Mia didn't return your call?** S: **Perhaps she didn't get the message or was too busy or forgot to call.**
28. Practices good sportsmanship.	SLP: **Let's talk about some ways to show good sportsmanship after a game.** S: **Congratulate the winner. If we win, we can accept congratulations in a friendly way. Say, "Good game!"**

(continues)

Objectives	Examples
29. Accepts "no" for an answer graciously and goes on to other activities.	SLP: **How can we accept it when a teacher or a friend says "no"?** S: **We can say "okay" in a friendly way without begging or pouting, then find other things to do.**
30. Firmly says "no" to unreasonable or harmful requests of others.	SLP: **At times everyone needs to say "no" if "yes" would result in trouble. Take Mary, for example. Mary's older cousin Dana pulled out a pack of cigarettes and said, "I'll teach you to smoke after our parents leave." Mary knew that cigarettes cause cancer and other diseases she didn't want. How could she say "no"?** S: **She could say, "Hey, cigarette smoking is not for me. I won't be smoking with you."**
31. Finds mutually acceptable solutions to conflicts with peers and adults.	SLP: **Did you like the video about handling disagreements? Tell us the most important thing you learned.** S: **Talking is important. Solutions come only when everyone in the conflict gets together to talk. They must be honest and courteous.**

Classroom Communication Skills

Yearly Goal: *To use communication skills to communicate and respond in styles appropriate to situations and listeners within the classroom environment*

CCSS.ELA-LITERACY.RL.2.6
CCSS.ELA-LITERACY.SL.K.1.A–3.1.A
CCSS.ELA-LITERACY.SL.4.1.B–SL.5.1.B
CCSS.ELA-LITERACY.SL.4.1.C–SL.8.1.C
CCSS.ELA-LITERACY.SL.K.2 and SL.1.2
CCSS.ELA-LITERACY.SL.2.3
CCSS.ELA-LITERACY.SL.3.1.C
CCSS.ELA-LITERACY.SL.3.3
CCSS.ELA-LITERACY.W.3.4–W.5.4

Objectives	Examples
Short-Term Goal: Knows and follows classroom communication routines	
1. Talks at appropriate times.	SLP: **Let's list some times you should and should not talk in the classroom.** S: **Should: Group discussion, free time, answering a teacher's question.** **Should not: During a test, in silent reading time, when the teacher is talking.**

Objectives	Examples
2. Waits for recognition before talking in class.	SLP: **How can you get the teacher's attention before you talk in class?** S: **Raise my hand and wait to be called on.**
3. Uses politeness markers.	SLP: **This bag has cards with polite words and phrases in it, such as *please, thank you, may I,* and *excuse me*. Pick a card and then use it correctly.** S: Chooses *excuse me* and says, **Excuse me, are you in this line?**
4. Changes communication style depending on the listener and the situation.	SLP: **Suppose you and your friends are talking casually in a group. How might your communication style change if an adult joins your group?** S: **With friends I might say, "No way, Jeff." With the adult, I would use a more formal style, such as, "I don't believe so, Mr. Baldridge."**
Short-Term Goal: Asks and answers questions	
5. Answers or attempts to answer questions when called on in class and to continue a conversation.	SLP: **What should you do if the teacher calls on you to answer a question or if a friend asks a question during a conversation?** S: **Try my best to answer it and stay on topic.**
6. Asks questions appropriate to the conversation or discussion to gain information or to clarify comprehension.	SLP: **Let's say you are in a discussion about Alaska and you want to know more about it. What kinds of questions could you ask?** S: **A question about the topic of conversation, a question to gain more information, and a question to clarify something I don't understand.**
Short-Term Goal: Participates in classroom discussions	
7. Uses tone of voice and loudness appropriate to the situation.	SLP: **Look at these pictures of different speaking situations. Say the sentence "Let's talk about it tomorrow" in the tone of voice and loudness that fits the situation.** S: Adjusts tone of voice and loudness to match the library, the playground, a small group, a large group, and talking to a friend on the bus.
8. Makes on-topic remarks that are brief and to the point.	SLP: **List some good ways to participate in a discussion.** S: **Listen to the topic being discussed, and make a brief remark to continue the topic. Try not to be the one who does all of the talking.**

(continues)

Objectives	Examples
9. Expresses and provides reasons for opinions in discussions.	SLP: **Sometimes it's good to give your opinions in a discussion. When you do, it's important that the listener knows it's an opinion and not a fact. Tell me an opinion and a fact for why you don't like to fly.** S: **Opinion: Flying is for the birds.** **Fact: I don't like to fly because it makes me sick.**
Short-Term Goal: Performs before others	
10. Participates in a role-playing activity.	SLP: **Role play can make a character come to life for you as you become that person. Role-play Meg's response in *A Wrinkle in Time* when Meg first sees her little brother, Charles Wallace, after their dangerous separation. How will Meg show her love for him?** S: **I'll show Meg's feelings in my voice. "I love you, Charles Wallace. You are the light of my life and treasure of my heart!"**
11. Reads aloud in front of a small group.	SLP: **Are you ready to make this story come alive for your audience? You can do that as you read this passage. Make your audience see and hear Granpa. Take on Granpa's voice in *The Education of Little Tree*.** S: (reads) **"Granpa said if you showed a feller how to do, it was a lot better than giving him something. He said if you learnt a man to make it for hisself, then he would be all right."**
12. Gives a report or makes a presentation in front of the class.	SLP: **Are you ready to give your report about the artist Georgia O'Keefe? Be sure to speak clearly with good volume.** S: **Georgia O'Keefe showed great talent from childhood. A famous photographer noticed her art and showed it in exhibits around the world. Thousands came and appreciated her art.**
Short-Term Goal: Follows oral instructions	
13. Follows oral instructions exactly.	SLP: **In class, you need to follow your teacher's instructions exactly. Let's try one: Write your last name in the top left corner.** S: Follows the directions correctly.

Objectives	Examples
14. Asks for clarification when instructions are unclear.	SLP: **What should you do if you don't understand the teacher's directions? Give an example.** S: I need to realize that I don't understand and then ask a question to make it clear. An example is "I'm not sure. Did you want me to take this note to Mr. Reyes or Mr. Gentry?"
Short-Term Goal: Gives spoken instructions	
15. Clearly names or describes objects and locations when giving instructions.	SLP: **Today will be fun. You get to play a barrier game with a partner. Your partner must hear clear instructions from you. Tell him how to arrange three objects: tree, house, person. Then give your partner a turn to instruct you.** S: (instructs a partner) Put the house to the left of the tree and the person to the right of the tree.
16. Watches the listener's reactions to check for understanding.	SLP: **During a conversation, certain clues let you know if your partner understands you. Ask yourself, "Did Matt seem to understand me?" How will you suspect that he didn't understand?** S: He had a confused look on his face, or there were restless body movements, or he kept looking at the clock.
17. Changes the instructions when the listener doesn't seem to understand by repeating or rephrasing without blaming the listener.	SLP: **Suppose your friend Lola seems confused. You just said, "Leave your notebook with her." What information could you add in a friendly way?** S: I could say politely, "Leave it with Mrs. Nibling, the school secretary."
Short-Term Goal: Follows written instructions	
18. Reads the entire sequence of instructions before beginning work or asking a question.	SLP: **Does your teacher sometimes give you written instructions only? What do you need to remember at those times? Why?** S: Read all the instructions to find out what to do. That way, if I need to ask a question, I'll know exactly what information to ask for.
19. Reads and explains written instructions in the correct sequence.	SLP: **Do you love to drink chocolate milk? Yum! Read and explain in your own words the steps in this recipe for making chocolate milk.** S: To make chocolate milk, get a glass, a carton of milk, and some chocolate syrup. Pour the syrup into the glass, add the milk, stir it up, and then enjoy!

(*continues*)

Objectives	Examples
Short-Term Goal: Gives clear written instructions	
20. States the overall objective in one sentence.	SLP: **When you get written instructions, do you like to know the main idea? Let's practice. Explain in writing the most important idea to know before planting flower seeds.** S: (writes) Before you plant the seeds, it's important to know how much sunlight flowers will need and how deeply to plant the seed.
21. Uses clear, short sentences to convey an idea.	SLP: **I want you to write instructions for making toast. Be sure to write clear, short sentences.** S: (writes) Set out a toaster, plate, butter, and two slices of bread. Plug in the toaster. Put the bread in the toaster. Turn it on. When the toast pops up, put the toast on the plate. Spread butter on the hot toast. Enjoy!
22. Gives the appropriate amount of information.	SLP: **It can be confusing to get too much information when you read instructions. Give enough information but not too much. For a partner, write instructions about how to get to the library from our classroom.** S: (writes) Go out the classroom door and turn right. Walk to the end of the hall. Turn left. The library is the first room on your right.

Classroom Social Survival Skills

Yearly Goal: *To use appropriate classroom social survival skills to understand and follow rules for expected behavior in the classroom and school environment*

CCSS.ELA-LITERACY.SL.K.2–SL.1.2
CCSS.ELA-LITERACY.SL.2.3
CCSS.ELA-LITERACY.SL.3.1.C

Objectives	Examples
Short-Term Goal: Accepts authority and interacts appropriately with teachers	
1. Complies with teacher requests.	SLP: **What should you do when the teacher asks you to do something?** S: **Do what she asks in a friendly, polite manner.**

Objectives	Examples
2. Knows and follows the classroom rules and classroom routine, regardless of whether the teacher is present.	SLP: **Every classroom has rules. How can you remember your classroom rules? What should students do?** S: **Look at the poster in our room to remind us of the rules. We should follow the rules.**
3. Works quietly during tests and seat work.	SLP: **Why is it important to work quietly when the class is taking a test or doing seat work?** S: **So we won't bother others.**
4. Monitors own actions by understanding how to keep them appropriate to given tasks.	SLP: **There are reasons students must think about their actions in the classroom. What will the teacher think if you whisper during a test?** S: **That you are asking for or giving test answers.**
5. Knows when help is needed and asks for clarification of specific parts instead of asking for the entire directions to be repeated.	SLP: **When you don't understand something, try to ask about a specific part that's giving you trouble instead of saying "Huh?" or "I don't know what to do." Why is this true?** S: **The teacher can help you more quickly when you say exactly what you don't understand.**
Short-Term Goal: Shows good attending behaviors	
6. Looks at the teacher and gives appropriate eye contact when she is talking or giving instructions.	SLP: **I am going to show you some ways to let your teacher know that you are or are not listening. If I show that I'm listening, give me a thumbs-up. If it looks like I'm not listening, give me a thumbs-down.** SLP looks at pretend teacher, nods at the teacher, drops pencil on the floor, looks at a book, and so on. S: Shows thumbs-up or thumbs-down.
7. Listens to peers or guest presentations with good attending behaviors: 1. Use good eye contact. 2. Keep hands still. 3. Make brief comments or ask brief questions.	SLP: **To show the speaker that you are listening to her presentation, you can do things like use good eye contact, keep your hands still, and ask questions. Show us some good or bad attending behaviors, and we will guess if they are good or bad.** S: Takes turns exhibiting good and poor attending behaviors.
Short-Term Goal: Knows and follows school routines	
8. Stays in seat when expected to by the teacher.	SLP: **Why is it important for students to stay in their seats and not walk about the classroom without permission?** S: **It disturbs other students when students do not stay in their seats.**

(continues)

Objectives	Examples
9. Understands and follows the teachers' cues.	SLP: **It's important to learn when your teacher is changing to a new activity. Watch what I do, and tell me what it might mean.** SLP acts out teacher's cues, such as getting out a math book, writing directions on the board, and standing by the door with his lunch satchel. S: Tells what those actions might mean.
10. Works cooperatively on a task with a partner.	SLP: **Let's list some good and bad things to do when working with a partner. Tell me something about working with a partner. We will write poor behaviors on the left side of the board and good behaviors on the right side.** S: **Bad things to do: Do all of the work yourself, let your partner do all of the work, do all of the talking.** **Good things to do: Do your best work, take turns listening and speaking, listen to your partner's ideas.**
11. Participates appropriately with peers in games, sports, and recess activities.	SLP: **Draw a picture of a good way and a bad way to play with your friends during sports or recess.** S: Draws pictures or activities such as waiting for a turn or hitting someone with a ball.
Short-Term Goal: Stays on task	
12. Avoids distracting others.	SLP: **What are some things you should not do so that you won't bother other people?** S: **Make noises, move a lot, drum your fingers on desks, or talk about other things.**
13. Ignores distractions of others or distractions in the environment.	SLP: **What should you do if other students are keeping you from working by talking or making noises?** S: **I need to ignore them and remind myself to keep working.**
14. Informs the teacher when having difficulty concentrating.	SLP: **Students must be able to concentrate in the classroom. What should you do when a nearby classmate is consistently disruptive?** S: **Let the teacher know and ask to be moved to a different seat.**
15. Works steadily for the required length of time.	SLP: **Can you give yourself tips to help you keep attending and working steadily?** S: **Set myself a timer for how many minutes I plan to work on an assignment. Tell myself, "Keep working. Don't stop."**

Objectives	Examples
16. Changes from one lesson or activity on the schedule to another.	SLP: **Teachers give signals that they are about to wrap up a lesson. How can you keep on attending while a teacher is wrapping up a lesson?** S: **Don't put things away until he finishes. Tell myself, "Focus. Don't stop listening."**
17. Completes academic work.	SLP: **What can you tell yourself to be sure you finish your work?** S: **Don't give up. Keep working. Pay attention to the work until it is finished.**
Short-Term Goal: Produces work acceptable to ability level	
18. Turns in neat papers.	SLP: **Let's look at your work. I want you to put a green check mark on the ones that are nice and neat and put a red check mark on the ones that could be better. What could you do to make the red-checked papers into green-checked ones?** S: Monitors the appearance of his work. **I could work more slowly and carefully.**
19. Accepts a teacher's correction of schoolwork.	SLP: **I want you to pretend to be my teacher and suggest ways to improve a paper or project. Give me a thumbs-up if I accept the comments appropriately and a thumbs-down if I don't. (1) Thanks, I'll remember that next time. (2) I can't ever do anything right!** S: Thumbs-up. Thumbs-down.
20. Checks schoolwork for errors.	SLP: **What should you do before you turn in a completed paper or project?** S: **Look over it one more time to see if there are any errors I could correct.**
21. Monitors the quality of his performance.	SLP: **What are some questions you should ask yourself to be sure you are doing your best work?** S: **What is the task? Am I doing it? How well have I done it?**
Short-Term Goal: Accepts responsibility for learning	
22. Attempts to solve problems with schoolwork before asking for help.	SLP: **Raise your hand when I say the best thing to do when you come to something hard with your schoolwork: (1) Go to the teacher's desk and ask for help right away. (2) Throw your paper on the floor and give up. (3) Give yourself a little more time to think about the task before asking for help.** S: Raises hand for (3).

(continues)

Objectives	Examples
23. Knows how to associate new information with information previously learned.	SLP: **When a new idea is presented, you should try to associate it with something you already know. Let's try one. What could you ask yourself when you are about to read a new story that takes place in Africa?** S: **What do I already know about Africa that will help me understand this new story?**
24. Finds acceptable use of time while waiting for teacher assistance.	SLP: **Let's pretend that you need your teacher's help with one math problem. Act out what you could do, and we will decide if that's a good way to wait for help.** S: Takes turns acting out good and poor ways to wait, such as calling the teacher's name over and over, taking a nap, working on another math problem, waiving a hand in the air, and trying the problem again.
25. Finds acceptable use of free time when work is completed.	SLP: **Tell me some things you should and should not do if you finish your work early. I'll write them on the board.** S: **Good: Read a library book, catch up on other work, check my assignment for any errors.** **Poor: Talk to my neighbor, get up and run around the room.**

Narrative Discourse

Yearly Goal: *To use the framework of narrative discourse to comprehend and structure age-appropriate oral or written narratives*

CCSS.ELA-LITERACY.RL.K.2–RL.8.2
CCSS.ELA-LITERACY.RL.1.4–RL.5.4
CCSS.ELA-LITERACY.RL.K.3–RL.4.3 and RL.6.3 and RL.8.3
CCSS.ELA-LITERACY.SL.2.2–SL.8.2

Note: Please see Appendix B ("Word Lists") for a list of conjunctions and transition words. See the visual organizers in Appendix C for a story map, episode map, and simple causal narrative map to help in planning intervention with these objectives.

Objectives	Examples
Short-Term Goal: Develops basic narrative abilities: Preschool–Grade 3	
1. Listens for increasingly longer time periods to stories appropriate to age level and responds to the storyteller's questions and requests by pointing to pictures.	SLP: **Did you like the story *Pancakes for Breakfast*? Look at the picture. Point to the eggs.**

Objectives	Examples
2. Acts out simple scripts about familiar events (e.g., going to the doctor, getting a haircut, going to school, eating breakfast).	SLP: **I need your help. I've been invited to a birthday party. I'm a little worried because I haven't been to one. I don't know what happens at a birthday party. Use these toys to show me what happens.** S: Acts out bringing a present, blowing out candles, singing "Happy Birthday," and so on.
3. Retells a personal experience while looking at pictures about it (photos or drawings) or telling about an object that represents the experience (souvenir).	SLP: **Here are three pictures about things we did on a trip to the zoo. Tell about them.** S: **In this one, we're getting on the bus that took us to the zoo. This one shows the monkeys we saw. The last one shows us eating lunch under a big tree at the zoo.**
4. Participates in a simple role play (one interaction) by taking the role of one of the characters in stories that have been read aloud.	SLP: **Let's pretend to be people in the story of *Pancakes for Breakfast*. I'll be the woman who makes the pancakes. I'll say, "My pancakes need syrup."** S: **I'll be the man who sells syrup. I'll say, "Would you like to buy some syrup?"**
5. Through role play demonstrates an understanding of episodes, sequences, settings, and characters in a predictable story, such as *The Three Pigs*, after hearing it several times.	SLP: **Let's act out the story of *The Three Billy Goats Gruff*. Would you like to be the Troll? What will you say each time a billy goat tramps across your bridge? What kind of voice will you use?** S: **I'll say, "WHO'S THAT TRAMPING ON MY BRIDGE?"**
6. Reorders picture scenes that have been scrambled and tells the story.	SLP: **Let's tell stories about visiting the dentist. Put these picture scenes in the right order and tell the story.** S: **(1) I say hello to the dentist. (2) I sit in the dental chair. (3) I lean back and open my mouth. (4) The dentist checks my teeth.**
7. Describes a pictured activity scene, such as going on a field trip, by telling the setting, theme, some details, reasons, and outcomes or predictions: 1. Setting: last week in the school parking lot 2. Theme: going on a field trip 3. Some details: wearing jackets and carrying sack lunches 4. Reasons: We look happy because we are having fun. 5. Outcomes: Everyone hopes to take another field trip.	SLP: **Here is a picture about our field trip. Tell about the setting and what's happening.** S: **The setting is the school parking lot last week. The bus driver is waiting for our class to get on the bus. We're getting on the bus. It's a cool day, so we have jackets on. We're carrying sack lunches. Everyone looks happy because we're having fun. Everyone hopes we go again!**

(continues)

Objectives	Examples
8. Listens to a familiar story in which an important episode has been omitted and then tells the omitted episode.	SLP: **We have read the story of *The Little Red Hen* many times. Listen carefully because this time when I read the story, I will leave out one important part. After the story, tell the part that I left out.** S: **You left out the part when Little Red Hen watered the seed.**
9. While looking at pictures, retells one essential part of a simple episode: 1. Setting: who, what, where, when 2. Initiating event: the beginning event 3. Situation, problem 4. Attempt: what they did about the problem 5. Outcome or consequence: the result, solution, ending	SLP: **Let's look at these sequence pictures of *The Little Red Hen* story. Samuel, retell the part that your picture shows.** S: **Little Red Hen said, "Who will help me plant the seed?" Every animal said, "Not I. I will not help you plant the seed." She said, "Then I will plant the seed myself." And she did.**
10. Tells or retells a simple one-episode story that includes four essentials while looking at cue cards or pictures: 1. Setting: who, what, where, when 2. Initiating event: beginning, situation, problem 3. Attempt: what the character did about it 4. Outcome: the result, solution, ending	SLP: **Each of you will take a turn retelling part of the story *Seymour's Problem* while looking at a picture.** S1: **Here is Seymour in his seat in his classroom.** S2: **Seymour forgot his school lunch box.** S3: **He felt embarrassed and worried.** S4: **Finally, Seymour told his teacher. She said, "You may have a lunch pass today."** S5: **Seymour felt happy while eating with friends.**
11. Retells one complete episode within a multi-episode story with the assistance of pictures and an episode map, story map, or flow chart. *Note:* Refer to the episode map in Appendix C for visual organizers.	SLP: **Today we will use an episode map to organize the story *The Show-and-Tell Frog*. Let's finish it together. Mia, please retell the first episode.** S: Using the episode map: **Alice lost her show-and-tell frog. She looked and looked, but she couldn't find it. She had to leave for school. She didn't see her little frog jump into her backpack. She felt terrible.**
Short-Term Goal: Develops advanced narrative abilities: Grades 3–8	
12. Defines key words before reading the story.	SLP: **Before we read *Too Many Tamales* by Gary Soto, let's define some important words from the story. Match these words to their definitions on the board: *masa* and *knead*.** S: ***Masa* is dough made from corn flour used to make tortillas and tamales. *Knead* means to squeeze dough with your hands to get it ready to bake.**

Objectives	Examples
13. Describes the characters' feelings and explains reasons for them.	SLP: **In the story, Maria's feelings changed often. Take turns telling three ways Maria felt at different times in the story, and tell the reasons.** S1: **Maria felt proud and grown up when she helped her mother make masa because she knew she was able to help.** S2: **Maria felt wishful when she looked at her mother's ring because she thought it was beautiful.** S3: **Maria felt shocked and sad when she discovered the ring was gone. She knew it was her fault that it was lost.**
14. Tells or retells a complete story that contains two to three episodes with the assistance of pictures and an episode map, story map, or flow chart. *Note:* Refer to the episode map in Appendix C for visual organizers.	SLP: **Use your episode map to help you organize and retell *Too Many Tamales*. Include a beginning, two or three episodes, and a clear ending.** S1: **Episode 1: Maria helped her mother make masa. She longed to wear her mother's pretty ring. She took it when her mother wasn't looking, but she planned to bring it back.** S2: **Episode 2: Maria finished the masa, but she forgot about the ring. She didn't know it had slipped off her finger.** S3: **Episode 3: Her cousins came. Maria noticed the ring was gone. Could it be in a tamale? Her cousins looked for it by eating all the tamales.** S4: **Episode 4: Nobody found the ring. Maria told her mother she had taken it. She felt very sorry.** S5: **Conclusion: Mother had found her ring earlier. Maria felt relieved. Everyone was happy and started making more tamales!**
15. While telling or retelling a story, uses appropriate connecting words that lend cohesion and show an understanding of the sequence and relationships within the story.	SLP: **Retell *Too Many Tamales* again but use at least two connecting words, such as *then, because, while, after, before that, later, finally*.** S: ***After* the cousins came, Maria noticed the ring was gone. She felt terrible. Could it be in a tamale? To look for the ring, the cousins ate all the tamales. *Before that*, the mom had found the ring herself. Maria was relieved. *Then* they made more tamales.**
16. Introduces two major characters appropriately when telling or retelling a story, giving information such as appearance, age, gender, and likes or dislikes.	SLP: **We read the book *Amazing Grace* by Mary Hoffman and Caroline Binch. How shall we describe Grace? Think about her age, likes or dislikes, appearance, and gender.** S: **Grace was an African American girl who loved stories of all kinds. She believed in herself.**

(*continues*)

Objectives	Examples
17. Identifies the effect of the characters' feelings and motivations on the events and the effect of the events on the characters' feelings and motivations.	SLP: **We finished our book *April Morning* by Howard Fast. Explain how Adam's terror during the battle affected his life.** S: **During the battle, Adam's reaction showed that he was only a boy. He was horrified. He screamed and ran away. He was able, however, to return. After the battle, Adam had changed from a boy to a man. He was able to take responsibility for his family at a young age.**
18. Dramatizes imaginary experiences that include the following: 1. Purpose: the event and internal response 2. Attempts to solve the problem 3. Internal responses: feelings 4. Direct consequences of the attempts *Note:* Refer to the story grammar components and simple causal narrative map in the visual organizers in Appendix C.	SLP: **Today we will work together again to plan a short play. Yesterday you decided to make the play about space travelers who land on a planet infested by a forest of meat-eating trees. They must pass through that land to find water.** S: Students work together to plan the story.
19. Rewrites stories into plays and participates in the enactment of them. Plan these areas: 1. Setting 2. Feelings 3. Characters' motivations 4. Structure of the episodes (acts) 5. Consequences of characters' actions 6. Outcome	SLP: **On the basis of your reading of the book *Island of the Blue Dolphins*, you will form teams to discuss and rewrite part of a chapter into a play. Plan the setting, the characters' feelings and motivations, the structure of the episodes (acts), the consequences of characters' actions, and the outcome.** S: Several students work together to rewrite a story.
20. Tells or helps write an original story that includes three episodes, connecting words, and the story grammar components. *Note:* See the basic story grammar components in Appendix C.	SLP: **This week we will work in teams to create an original story. It will include three episodes and the story grammar components that are shown on the chart. Include connecting and transition words to help your story flow smoothly.** S: Students work together to create a story and share it.

Unit 2

Vocabulary and Meaning

- Labels and Categories
- Action and Function Concepts: Verbs
- Quality Concepts: Adjectives
- Position and Time Concepts: Prepositions
- Answering Questions
- Formulating Definitions
- Comparing and Contrasting Meanings
- Antonyms
- Synonyms
- Multiple-Meaning Words
- Homonyms
- Word Relationships
- Verbal Analogies
- Figurative Language
- Inferences, Predictions, and Outcomes

A child's understanding of word meaning is dependent on his or her underlying concepts and knowledge of the world (Owens, 2010). *Meaning* consists of concepts that extend beyond the word level. A *concept* is an idea that combines several elements from different sources into a single notion. These ideas or meanings are usually mediated by a word, symbol, or sign. Various words and phrases modify meanings through their syntactic arrangement, shades of meaning, speaker or writer intents, and word relationships.

Planning for the development of vocabulary and meaning demands expertise in teaching concepts. Hands-on, interactive experiences, especially for young children, are widely acknowledged to be the best context for teaching vocabulary. It is important to teach a concept in a variety of ways. For example, when you are teaching the concepts of *first* and *last*, let the child experience being first and last in line or racing toy cars to see which ones come in first and last. Talk about the first and last days of the month, sounds in a word, and steps in making a craft. The child should be able to use and understand the concept with actions, objects, and pictures; on a work sheet; and in writing. Use of role play, objects, and real-life situations enhances the learning experience. Older children have a burst of concept development when they begin to read. They add exponentially to their concept knowledge through reading. All children gain word meaning vicariously by discussing what they have read or experienced with others.

There are several things to consider when choosing which words to teach in order to build a child's vocabulary. The number of words in a child's vocabulary is not the only factor to be considered. Diversity in types of words is also important. Attention to teaching verbs, adjectives, and prepositions is just as important as building a child's knowledge of nouns. Adult clarification about words, especially when reading, is also essential (Schuele, 2011). According to Beck, McKeown, and Kucan (2003), not all words are created equal. Words can be divided into Tier 1 (everyday words, such as *book* and *run*), Tier 2 (more specific words, such as *novel* and *sprint*), and Tier 3 (domain-specific words, such as *syntax* and *velars*). Most children are exposed to Tier 1 words, but children who need vocabulary development benefit from intentional teaching of higher level Tier 2 words.

The speech–language pathologist (SLP) and classroom teacher compose the perfect team to increase the understanding of concepts within the student's experiences at school. This unit provides objectives to aid program planning for students who need to develop vocabulary and meaning. These objectives help the SLP and classroom teacher plan individualized lessons for improving not only basic word knowledge in young children but also higher level concepts in older students. Such goals include understanding and using word relationships, comparing and contrasting meanings, understanding inferences, and making predictions.

During lesson planning, several parts of this unit may be linked effectively to objectives in other units. For example, objectives for students in Grades 2–12 who are working on understanding inferences and other implied meanings can be used with objectives in Reading Comprehension of Literature: Grades 4–8 (pp. 142–145). Reading comprehension can also be enhanced by objectives in Comparing and Contrasting Meanings (pp. 49–51) and Multiple-Meaning Words (pp. 54–55) in this unit. For help in planning intervention using the objectives in this unit, see Appendix A, "First Words" (pp. 209–210), and Appendix B, "Word Lists" (Labels and Categories, Position Concepts [Prepositions], Quality Concepts [Adjectives], Temporal Concepts, Antonyms, Synonyms, Multiple-Meaning Words, Homonyms, Verbal Analogies, and Figurative Language) (pp. 211–220).

Labels and Categories

Yearly Goal: *To develop vocabulary by naming and categorizing objects, pictures, and ideas*

CCSS.ELA-LITERACY.L.K.5.A–L.1.5.A

Note: See Appendix B ("Word Lists") for lists of labels and categories.

Objectives	Examples
1. Understands and says words to label familiar toys, foods, clothes, objects, activities, actions, and body parts.	SLP: **Let's find your favorite toys and say their names. Next, tell me some of the clothes you are wearing today.** S: **Truck, bear, blocks; shirt, pants, shoes**
2. Understands and says words to label familiar words and concepts, such as vehicles, buildings, household items, tools, holidays, and sports.	SLP: **Drive your toy car around the town. Name the places, things, and people you pass.** S: **Store, school, hospital, fire truck, train, doctor, boy, police officer**
3. Names three selected pictures from a given category.	SLP: **Name these vehicles we are playing with.** S: **Boat, ambulance, school bus**
4. Chooses an object or picture to match a given category.	SLP: **Show me the musical instrument. Point to an animal.** S: Shows a trumpet and points to a bear.
5. Sorts objects or pictures into two categories.	SLP: **Let's pretend we work in a grocery store and divide this toy food into fruits and vegetables.** S: Sorts fruits (apples, bananas, and grapes) and vegetables (carrots, green beans, and corn).
6. Groups objects or pictures by given category descriptions or names.	SLP: **On this work sheet, circle all the things you can eat. Put an X on the things you can ride.** S: Puts an X on the bike and bus, and circles the sandwich and cookie.
7. Categorizes objects or pictures by attributes.	SLP: **Let's pretend we are at the grocery store. Put the sweet foods in the cart. Give me the foods that are red.** S: Puts candy and cake in the cart, and gives the SLP a strawberry and an apple.
8. Names a category to describe a set of objects or pictures.	SLP: **Look at these pictures. What group do the truck, boat, and car belong to?** S: **Vehicles**
9. Finds the object, picture, or word that does not belong in a given category.	SLP: **On this activity sheet, underline the animal that does not belong: parrot, robin, turtle.** S: (underlines) turtle

(continues)

Objectives	Examples
10. Names the category to which a spoken word belongs.	SLP: **What group does a dog belong to? Name a category for these words: *piano, guitar, violin.*** S: **Animals, musical instruments**
11. Names multiple items of a given category.	SLP: **Let's brainstorm together and try to name all of the jungle animals we can think of.** S: **Lion, tiger, giraffe**
12. Names an item when given its category and description.	SLP: **Guess what I am talking about. It's a fruit. It's long and yellow and you peel it.** S: **A banana**
13. Describes a category by listing some of its functions or attributes.	SLP: **We are going to divide into two groups. Tell some things about the category I whisper to you, and your friends will guess what it is.** SLP whispers "vehicles." S: **They move. People can ride in or on them. Some of them have wheels.**
14. Tells how two objects, pictures, or events from the same category are different.	SLP: **Choose two fruits from this bag. How are they different?** S: **The cherry is small, red, and sweet; the lemon is larger, yellow, and sour.**
15. Tells how two objects, pictures, or events from the same category are alike.	SLP: **Choose two picture cards from this stack. Tell me some ways they are the same.** S: **The shirt and pants both are made from cloth and have buttons, and you wear them.**

Action and Function Concepts: Verbs

Yearly Goal: *To develop understanding and spontaneous use of action verbs in listening, speaking, reading, and writing*

CCSS.ELA-LITERACY.L.K.1.B
CCSS.ELA-LITERACY.L.K.5.B
CCSS.ELA-LITERACY.L.1.1.C
CCSS.ELA-LITERACY.L.K.5.D–L.1.5.D and L.2.5.B

Objectives	Examples
1. Uses a toy to demonstrate some actions of given verbs.	SLP: **Let's play a listening game with these toys. Choose a toy and make the toy do what I say: Bounce the ball.**
2. Demonstrates an action upon hearing a single verb.	SLP: **Show us what this word means by acting it out: *jump.***

Objectives	Examples
3. Demonstrates actions of given verbs in the third person using objects such as a doll or a toy bear.	SLP: **Choose a stuffed animal from the shelf. Now make it do what I say: He is waving. He is sitting. He is jumping.** S: Makes a toy bear wave, sit, and jump.
4. Points to the correct picture among a group of pictures showing a named motor activity.	SLP: **The children in these pictures are having fun. Point to the child who is running.**
5. Names demonstrated motor activities.	SLP: **Today you'll take turns acting out a word I whisper to you. What is Tom doing?** S: **Skipping**
6. Names pictured verbs.	SLP: **Let's look at what's happening in this story-book. What is this bear doing?** S: **Eating**
7. Follows verbal commands containing action verbs.	SLP: **Let's play Simon Says. Listen: Simon says, "Clap your hands."** S: Claps hands.
8. Demonstrates understanding of frequently occurring verbs by relating them to their opposites.	SLP: **Today we'll play an opposites game. Do the opposite of what I say: "Becca, shout your name."** S: (whispers) **Becca**
9. Uses a phrase or sentence to describe actions performed by self.	SLP: **I'll whisper an action for you to show us. Use a sentence to tell us what you are doing.** S: **I am hopping.**
10. Uses a phrase or sentence to describe actions performed by others.	SLP: **We'll divide into small groups for exercise. Afterward, we will talk about what each one did. What was Amy doing?** S: **Amy was stretching.**
11. Uses singular and plural nouns with matching verbs in basic sentences.	SLP: **Look at these sets of action pictures. Here the girl eats. Here all the girls _____.** S: **Eat**
12. Describes an object by telling what can be done with it.	SLP: **You will have a turn to tell us what you can do with your show-and-tell. What can you do with your soccer ball?** S: **I can bounce and kick my soccer ball.**
13. Lists two or more actions someone or something can do.	SLP: **Did you like the dog story? Let's look at the pictures. Tell us two things a dog can do.** S: **Bark and run**
14. Answers true-or-false questions involving action verbs.	SLP: **Let's talk about some things we have learned about birds. Answer "true" or "false." Most birds can swim.** S: **False**

(continues)

Objectives	Examples
15. Identifies same-category verbs, such as *run* and *walk*.	SLP: **Tell which actions are alike: eat, gobble, sleep.** S: **eat and gobble**
16. Answers exclusionary agent–action questions, such as "What can't trees do?"	SLP: **Listen carefully. Tell me something frogs can't do.** S: **Frogs can't talk.**
17. Compares action–agent differences.	SLP: **Tell me what birds do that fish don't.** S: **Fish don't fly.**
18. Uses a verb correctly in a sentence.	SLP: **Read the verbs from your science lesson. Use the verb *melt* in a sentence.** S: **Snow melts when the sun comes out.**
19. Acts out shades of meaning among verbs expressing the same general action, such as *run*, *rush*, *hurry*, *race*.	SLP: **Act out the differences among these words: *wash, scrub, bathe*.**
20. Distinguishes shades of meaning among closely related verbs, such as *work*, *labor*, *toil*.	SLP: **Here are pictures of someone who falls, slips, trips, stumbles. Point to "The boy tripped" and "The boy slipped."**
21. Describes shades of meaning among verbs expressing the same general meanings, such as *throw*, *toss*, *pitch*.	SLP: **Tell the differences between these ways to gather flowers: pick, pull.** S: **To pick a flower, I quickly snap its stem. To pull a flower, I tug it out of the ground.**
22. Uses verbs correctly while retelling a story.	SLP: **Did you like the story of the *Mayflower*? Retell the story in your own words. Use these verbs: *sailed, landed, built, ate*.** S: **The *Mayflower* sailed from Spain. It landed on what we now call Plymouth Rock.**
23. Writes a verb correctly in a sentence.	SLP: **Use the verb *vote* in a sentence.** S: (writes) Today we vote for our favorite story.
24. Writes a set of related verbs correctly in a story.	SLP: **Today we will write a story about Thanksgiving together, and we'll use these verbs: *cook, carve, eat, feast*.** S: **Mom will cook a turkey, and Grandpa will carve it.**

Quality Concepts: Adjectives

Yearly Goal: *To develop vocabulary through understanding and spontaneous use of adjectives while listening, speaking, reading, and writing*

CCSS.ELA-LITERACY.L.1.1.F
CCSS.ELA-LITERACY.L.K.5.B
CCSS.ELA-LITERACY.L.1.5.D and L.2.5.B
CCSS.ELA-LITERACY.L.4.1.D
CCSS.ELA-LITERACY.L.2.6

Note: See Appendix B ("Word Lists") for lists of qualities.

Objectives	Examples
1. Chooses the object or picture described by one attribute.	SLP: **Here are some objects we've studied: airplane, train, bike. Which ones are noisy?** S: **The airplane and the train**
2. Uses the correct adjective to answer a question about the color, size, shape, number, or texture of an object.	SLP: **What shape is this tent?** S: **Triangle**
3. Chooses the object or picture described by two attributes.	SLP: **Look at the pictures of a lemon and a banana. Which one is long and yellow?** S: **The banana**
4. Names an object described by one attribute.	SLP: **Think of the fruits we've studied. Which ones are purple?** S: **Grapes and plums**
5. Names an object described by two attributes.	SLP: **Let's look at these foods we could eat for snack. Tell which food is both salty and crunchy.** S: **Pretzels**
6. Demonstrates understanding of frequently occurring adjectives by relating them to their opposites.	SLP: **Here are some weather pictures. Choose a picture that shows the opposite of what I say: It was a sunny day.** S: Chooses a rainy-day picture.
7. Answers true-or-false statements about attributes of objects or pictures.	SLP: **Look at these pictures from the story we just read and answer my question. True or false? The blocks are round.** S: **False**
8. Chooses the correct picture or names an object to answer exclusionary agent–action questions.	SLP: **Let's look at all of these weather pictures. Now find the picture of weather that is not stormy.** S: Points to the sunny picture.

(continues)

Objectives	Examples
9. Names multiple objects that a given attribute could describe.	SLP: **Tell me all the animals we've studied that are fast.** S: **Antelopes, deer, and tigers**
10. Distinguishes shades of meaning among adjectives that differ in intensity, such as *wee, teensy, tiny, small, little*.	SLP: **This work sheet from our book has pictures of pretend houses that bugs could live in. Circle the wee house of the flea and underline the small house of the ladybug.**
11. Names multiple objects that two given attributes could describe.	SLP: **Tell me all the fruits and vegetables you can think of that can be red and round.** S: **Apple, tomato, cherry**
12. Names objects an exclusionary attribute could describe.	SLP: **Look at all of these shapes. Name the shapes that don't have three corners.** S: **Circles, squares, rectangles, and hexagons**
13. Tells how two objects are alike or different using critical attributes.	SLP: **Think about all of the kinds of weather we have been learning about. How are rain and snow alike and different?** S: **Both are wet. They come from the sky. Snow is always cold, but rain is sometimes warm.**
14. Acts out shades of meaning among closely related adjectives, such as *quiet, silent, hushed, still, peaceful*.	SLP: **Think about the book we just finished. Act out the differences among these good ways the boy felt during his birthday party: pleased, cheerful, delighted.** S: Acts pleased when welcoming guests to the party and delighted when opening a present.
15. Matches written nouns in one list with their attributes in another list.	SLP: **Here is a list of nouns and another list of words that describe them. Draw a line to connect the label with its describing word.** S: Connects *elephant* with *huge*.
16. Writes an antonym or synonym for each adjective on a list.	SLP: **Write the opposite of *enormous*.** S: (writes) tiny
17. Orders adjectives within sentences according to conventional patterns.	SLP: **Write a sentence using two or three adjectives to describe an animal we saw on our nature walk.** S: (writes) We saw feisty little brown squirrels in the park.
18. Given a sentence or paragraph, modifies its meaning by adding or substituting adjectives.	SLP: **Add or substitute adjectives to change the meaning of this sentence: The little boy read his book in the library.** S: (writes) The curious boy read his nature book in the quiet library.
19. Uses critical attributes to write a definition of a given word.	SLP: **Use adjectives when you write a definition for the word *path*.** S: (writes) A path is a narrow walkway packed down by footsteps.

Position and Time Concepts: Prepositions

Yearly Goal: *To develop understanding and spontaneous use of prepositions in listening, speaking, reading, and writing*

CCSS.ELA-LITERACY.L.K.1.E and L.1.1.I
CCSS.ELA-LITERACY.L.4.1.E
CCSS.ELA-LITERACY.L.3.6
CCSS.ELA-LITERACY.W.1.3–W.2.3 and W.3.3.C

Note: See Appendix B ("Word Lists") for lists of location and time words.

Objectives	Examples
1. Points to an object in the position described.	SLP: **Point to the block under the book.**
2. Places self or an object in the position requested.	SLP: **Juan, please stand next to Paula.**
3. Points to the described picture that shows a position.	SLP: **Look at these pictures. Point to "The boy is behind the chair."**
4. Uses a single preposition to answer a question about a position.	SLP: **Let's play with these farm toys. Where is the cow?** S: **Behind**
5. Uses a single preposition to answer a question about time sequence.	SLP: **Think about our school day. When did we make our craft: after lunch or before lunch?** S: **After**
6. Answers a question using a prepositional phrase.	SLP: **I just read for you the story *Goldilocks and the Three Bears*. Use a phrase to answer my question. Where did Goldilocks go for a walk?** S: **In the woods**
7. Describes a picture using a preposition.	SLP: **Think about our science lesson about plants that we can eat. Tell me where a carrot grows.** S: **Under the ground**
8. Names the antonym or synonym of a given preposition.	SLP: **What's another word for *over*? What's the opposite of *before*?** S: **Above; after**
9. Uses prepositions to give oral directions about location.	SLP: **We are going to play a barrier game. Use some prepositions to tell your partner where to put the big block.** S: **Put the big block behind the little block.**
10. Uses prepositions to give oral directions about time.	SLP: **We are going to practice giving directions. Tell the students when to clap their hands.** S: **Clap your hands before you touch your knees.**

(continues)

Objectives	Examples
11. Using a pencil and paper, follows oral directions containing prepositions.	SLP: **On this work sheet, draw a circle between the tree and the flower.**
12. Writes a given preposition in a sentence or paragraph.	SLP: **Let's read this list of prepositions on the board. Now write the directions for building a birdhouse using these prepositions: *before, in, out, after, under.*** S: (writes) Before building a birdhouse, you need to get the materials. Be sure there is a hole in the birdhouse so that the birds can go in and out and so on.
13. Uses prepositions for location and time relations correctly in writing and speaking.	SLP: **When writing a report about your favorite trip and presenting it to the class, be sure to use some of the location and time words we have studied. Tell about the sequence of your trip from the time you left until you returned home.**

Answering Questions

Yearly Goal: *To improve understanding and the ability to answer* yes/no *and* wh- *questions while listening, speaking, reading, and writing*

CCSS.ELA-LITERACY.RI.K.1–2.1
CCSS.ELA-LITERACY.W.1.5
CCSS.ELA-LITERACY.SL.1.2

Teaching Note: An effective approach to teaching children to answer questions is to determine the lowest level of questions that the child can answer. Teach him or her to answer the next level and then work on those two question types combined. For example, teach *where*, then *when*, and then work on the two together.

Objectives	Examples
1. Answers *yes/no* questions that begin with *is, am, are, can, do, does.*	SLP: **Think about the food we have studied and answer these questions. Is an apple red? Do you eat cake for breakfast?** S: **Yes; no**
2. Answers *who* questions.	SLP: **Answer my questions while we walk around the school. Who works in the library? Who teaches PE?** S: **The librarian; Mr. Garcia**
3. Answers *what* questions with nouns.	SLP: **Look at the picture on this page. What is this boy wearing? What do you see in the tree?** S: **A coat; a bird**

Objectives	Examples
4. Answers *what* questions with verbs.	SLP: **Let's talk about your friends on the playground. What are they doing on the monkey bars? What is Don doing?** S: Climbing; Don is running.
5. Answers *what* questions with adjectives.	SLP: **We are going to have fun making this fruit salad. Let's look at this apple. What color is it? What shape is it? What size is it? What does it taste like?** S: Red; round; small; It tastes sweet.
6. Answers *where* questions.	SLP: **We have been studying about animals and their homes. Where does a bird live? Where can you find a whale?** S: In a nest; A whale is in the ocean.
7. Answers *yes/no* questions that begin with *will, would, shall, should, could, has, have, was, were.*	SLP: **I hope you liked the story of *Goldilocks and the Three Bears*. Should Goldilocks have gone into the three bears' house? Have you ever tasted porridge?** S: No; no
8. Answers *when* questions.	SLP: **Think about our school day schedule. When does school start? When do you eat lunch?** S: At 8:00; after our math lesson
9. Answers *how* questions.	SLP: **I like the work you did in art class. How did you make your picture? How do you feel when you are painting?** S: I colored it with chalk. I feel happy when I paint.
10. Answers *why* questions.	SLP: **Think about the science experiment we did yesterday. Why did we wear protective glasses? Why did we measure the liquid?** S: Because we needed to protect our eyes; so our experiment would work correctly
11. Answers *who, what, where, when, why,* and *how* questions about details in a text.	SLP: **We just read *The Very Hungry Caterpillar*. What did the caterpillar eat? When did he become a butterfly?** S: Pie, muffins, watermelon, and so on; when he came out of his cocoon
12. Writes answers to written questions.	SLP: **Read each question on this work sheet and write your answer.**
13. Writes a paragraph to answer all questions appropriately.	SLP: **Write a paragraph about today's Field Day and answer all of the questions on the board.**

Formulating Definitions

Yearly Goal: *To develop vocabulary and semantics through increasing ability to formulate word definitions while listening, speaking, and writing*

CCSS.ELA-LITERACY.L.1.5.B
CCSS.ELA-LITERACY.L.K.5.B
CCSS.ELA-LITERACY.L.4.5.C

Objectives	Examples
Short-Term Goal: States single essential attributes of objects or pictures	
1. Says the name of a picture or object.	SLP: **Look at this picture from our jungle lesson and tell me the name of these animals.** S: **Zebra, elephant**
2. Tells an attribute to describe a picture or object.	SLP: **Tell me some words to describe the picture of the zebra and the elephant.** S: **Striped; huge**
3. States the action or function of a picture or object.	SLP: **Tell me what a zebra can do.** S: **A zebra can run.**
4. Tells about an object, person, or place that is related to a given picture or object.	SLP: **Tell me some places that go with a zebra and an elephant.** S: **Africa, zoo**
5. Names the category to which a picture or object belongs.	SLP: **Tell me the group or category name for a zebra and an elephant.** S: **Animals**
Short-Term Goal: Identifies or tells multiple essential attributes in a definition	
6. Matches an object or picture to a given definition.	SLP: **On this work sheet, circle the picture of a large, furry animal that hibernates.** S: (circles) bear
7. Tells any two or three things about an object.	SLP: **Tell us two or three things about what you brought for show-and-tell.** S: **It's big and round and a toy.**
8. Tells at least three different things about a picture or object. These three could include the name; an attribute, action, or function; related objects, people, or places; and the category.	SLP: **Tell us three different things about this picture.** S: **A banana is a fruit. It's long and yellow and you eat it.**
9. Chooses the attributes of a pictured word.	SLP: **Circle the words on this work sheet that describe this picture of a strawberry.** S: (circles) red, sweet, small

Objectives	Examples
10. Matches attributes to associated words.	SLP: **Look at this list of vocabulary words and their attributes. Under the word *bird*, write the three words from the list that describe a bird.** S: (writes) wings, flies, beak
Short-Term Goal: Completes definitions with essential attributes	
11. Completes the definition for a pictured word.	SLP: **Read these geography definitions and look at the pictures. Name the picture that completes this definition: A body of land surrounded by water is called an _____.** S: **Island**
12. Completes a definition with its essential attributes.	SLP: **Finish this sentence: A shovel is a tool that is used for _____.** S: **Digging**
13. Chooses the most complete definition for a picture.	SLP: **Look at this picture of an artery from your science lesson. On the work sheet, circle the most complete definition. (1) A tube in the body with blood. (2) A tube in the body that carries blood away from the heart.** S: Circles the second definition.
Short-Term Goal: Forms definitions through the use of antonyms, synonyms, comparisons, and descriptors	
14. Demonstrates understanding of verbs and modifiers by stating antonyms of the words given.	SLP: **We are going to play charades. Act out the words I say, and your friends will guess the opposite: Stand up.** S1: Stands up. S2: **Sits down.**
15. Demonstrates understanding of nouns, verbs, and modifiers by stating synonyms of the words given.	SLP: **We are going to take turns building a block tower. Before you add your block to the tower, say a word that means the same as *car*.** S: **Automobile**
16. Defines modifiers by using the following: Comparisons: *Huge* means bigger than big. Synonyms: *Huge* means large. Descriptors: *Huge* means really big.	SLP: **Write definitions of *minuscule* using comparisons, synonyms, and descriptors.** S: (writes) *Minuscule* means smaller than small. *Minuscule* means tiny. *Minuscule* means very small.
17. Lists the critical attributes of a given definition.	SLP: **On this work sheet, underline the attributes that are critical to this definition and distinguish it from other definitions: A pair of scissors is a handheld cutting instrument with two blades whose cutting edges slide past each other.** S: (underlines) handheld, cutting, two blades

(continues)

Objectives	Examples
Short-Term Goal: Writes or tells definitions when given critical attributes	
18. Writes or states a definition using a list of given attributes.	SLP: **Use these words to write or tell a definition of *peninsula: land, water, three sides, connected.*** S: (writes or says) **A peninsula is a strip of land surrounded by water on three sides and connected to a larger body of land.**
19. Writes or states definitions of verbs by describing movements of associated objects.	SLP: **Write or tell the definition of *eating* by describing movements of associated objects.** S: (writes or says) **Eating is putting food in your mouth to chew and swallow.**
20. Writes or states definitions of objects by using modifiers, nouns, and verbs to describe critical features.	SLP: **Choose an object from this grab bag. Write or tell a definition of your object by describing its critical features with a modifier, noun, and verb.** S: (writes or says) **This ruler is a long, wooden (modifiers) tool that has numbers on it (nouns) and is used for measuring (verb).**
21. Writes or states definitions of nouns by using a category name and two critical attributes.	SLP: **Look at this picture from the social studies lesson. Write or tell the definition of a dime by using a category name and two critical attributes.** S: (writes or says) **A dime is a coin that is worth 10 cents and is used to buy things in the United States and Canada.**
22. Uses context to write definitions of selected words in a story.	SLP: **Use the context of this paragraph in your social studies book to write a definition of the word *freedom.*** S: (writes) Freedom is the right to act, speak, or think as one wants without being held back.

Comparing and Contrasting Meanings

Yearly Goal: *To compare and contrast meanings by developing understanding and use of similarities and differences between related words while listening, speaking, reading, and writing*

CCSS.ELA-LITERACY.L.K.5.A and L.1.5.A

Note: See the visual organizers in Appendix C for a sample compare–contrast concept map to use with these objectives.

Objectives	Examples
Short-Term Goal: Compares two related words by explaining their similarities	
1. Sorts common objects into categories to gain a sense of the concepts that the categories represent.	SLP: **Put these toy animals into two groups: farm animals and wild animals.** S: Farm animals: cow, pig, horse; wild animals: lion, elephant, zebra
2. Sorts words into categories to gain understanding of the concepts the categories represent.	SLP: **Read these cards. They have the names of clothing or the names of body parts. Put them in two groups: clothing and body parts.** S: Clothing: shirt, socks, hat; body parts: arm, head, toe
3. Names the category to tell how two words from the same category are similar.	SLP: **Let's talk about the food we used to make our snack. How are the apples and bananas alike? They are both _____.** S: **Fruits**
4. Names shared actions or functions (uses) to tell how two words are similar.	SLP: **I have a knife and some scissors. How are they alike? Tell about their uses.** S: **A knife and scissors are used to cut things.**
5. Names shared attributes (adjectives) and categories to tell how two words are similar.	SLP: **Here is some food we bought on our pretend grocery trip. Tell two ways these bananas and lemons are alike.** S: **Lemons and bananas are both fruits that are yellow and tasty.**
6. Names a shared space (location) to tell how two words are similar.	SLP: **Think about the bones in our bodies that we talked about in science class. Tell how these words are alike by their location: the fibula and the tibia.** S: **They are bones in our legs.**
7. Names a shared time (time words) to tell how two words are similar.	SLP: **In this weather book, we learned about sleet and snow. Compare sleet and snow by telling their category and a season.** S: **Snow and sleet are kinds of precipitation. They fall during winter.**

(continues)

Objectives	Examples
8. Names shared importance of two words to tell how they are similar.	SLP: **We learned a lot today during Career Day. Tell how these two occupations are similar by explaining their importance: education and nursing.** S: **Both occupations help people live better lives.**
Short-Term Goal: Contrasts two related words by explaining their differences	
9. Contrasts two subcategories to tell how two words from the same category are different.	SLP: **Think about the animals we have been studying. An elephant and alligator are both animals. Tell how they are different.** S: **An elephant is a mammal; an alligator is a reptile.**
10. Contrasts actions or functions (uses) to tell how two nouns are different.	SLP: **As we walked around the block today, we saw some light poles and some telephone poles. Tell how they are different by telling their uses.** S: **Light poles are used to hold streetlights, and telephone poles are used to hold telephone wires or cables.**
11. Contrasts critical attributes (adjectives) to tell how two nouns are different.	SLP: **Look at these pictures of fruits. Bananas and lemons are both fruits. Tell two important ways they are different.** S: **Lemons are oval shaped and taste sour: bananas are long and skinny and taste sweet.**
12. Contrasts two locations to tell how two nouns are different.	SLP: **Remember our discussion of animals and their homes. Include places or locations to tell how these animals are different: camels and penguins.** S: **Camels live in a hot desert; penguins live in Antarctica or other frigid areas.**
13. Contrasts two time words to tell how two nouns are different.	SLP: **Two types of weather we learned about are blizzards and hurricanes. Compare them and include seasons when each occurs.** S: **Blizzards come in winter, and hurricanes come in the fall.**
14. Gauges the importance of two items to tell how they are different.	SLP: **Compare the importance of the work of mail carriers and firefighters.** S: **Mail carriers help us send messages to one another; firefighters protect us from fires.**
Short-Term Goals: Defines synonyms by differentiating their similar qualities	
15. Writes two different sentences (one with each word) that show the similarities between the two words.	SLP: **Use synonyms to write similarities between hurricanes and blizzards.** S: (writes) A blizzard *destroyed* the Iowa farmland. A hurricane *demolished* buildings on the Atlantic coast.

Objectives	Examples
16. Writes two different sentences (one with each word) that show the differences between synonyms.	SLP: **Write two sentences about hurricanes and blizzards. In one sentence use *forceful*. In the other sentence use *powerful*.** S: (writes) *Forceful* freezing north winds of blizzards created freezing ice and snow that endangered cattle and people. *Powerful* tropical winds of hurricanes created high ocean waves that stormed the shoreline of the islands and endangered animals and people.
17. Writes or tells definitions of the words that have been compared.	SLP: **Define the words *blizzard* and *hurricane*.** S: (writes) A *blizzard* is a severe snowstorm with cold temperatures that leaves huge drifts of snow. A *hurricane* is powerful wind with high rainfall that happens near the ocean, especially the Atlantic.

Antonyms

Yearly Goal: *To develop understanding and spontaneous use of word opposites (antonyms) in listening, speaking, reading, and writing*

CCSS.ELA-LITERACY.L.K.5.B
CCSS.ELA-LITERACY.L.4.5.C and L.5.5.C

Note: See Appendix B ("Word Lists") for lists to help in planning with these objectives.

Objectives	Examples
1. Given a group of objects or pictures with opposite qualities, points to the one requested.	SLP: **Look at the pillow, rock, and book. Give me the soft one.** S: Picks up the pillow.
2. Matches a given picture with its opposite.	SLP: **Draw lines to match the opposites.** S: Draws a line between pictures of short and tall.
3. Describes objects or pictures with opposite qualities.	SLP: **Tell me how these two green blocks are different.** S: This block is big. That block is little.
4. Indicates whether two words have the same or different meanings.	SLP: **Give me a thumbs-up or thumbs-down sign. Show me if these two words have the same or different meanings: *tall, short*.** S: Shows thumbs-down.
5. When shown two pictures of opposite things and given a model sentence, responds with the opposite sentence.	SLP: **This animal hunts in the day. Tell me about the other picture.** S: That animal hunts at night.

(continues)

Objectives	Examples
6. Matches opposite words in different lists.	SLP: **On this page draw lines to match the opposites.** S: Matches the words *sorrow* and *joy*.
7. Says the appropriate opposite word to complete verbal analogies.	SLP: **Listen and tell me the correct opposite: To build up is to create. To tear down is to _____.** S: **destroy**
8. Says the opposite for a spoken word.	SLP: **Let's have an opposites bee. I'll say a word. Tell me the correct opposite word: *urban*.** S: **Rural**
9. Follows directions by doing the opposite, such as *look up*, *look down*.	SLP: **We'll play opposites charades. Group 1, you will act out the word I whisper to you: *bored*. Group 2, you will guess the opposite word.** S: **Interested**
10. Chooses the correct spoken word from an opposite pair to complete a sentence.	SLP: **Choose the correct word: You need to *arrive* or *depart* at the airport 2 hours before your flight.** S: **Arrive**
11. Writes the appropriate opposites in fill-in-the-blank sentences.	SLP: **Let's play an opposites game with words from the story we just read. Write the opposite word: In the beginning, the giants were rude. At the end the giants were _____.** S: (writes) polite
12. Corrects a written sentence or story by changing inappropriately used opposites.	SLP: **Correct this sentence by changing the incorrect opposite word: Turtles are among the world's swiftest animals.** S: (writes) slowest
13. Changes a written sentence or story by substituting opposites.	SLP: **Change the incorrect words by writing their opposites: Meredith wanted her letter to make a terrible impression on the boss. She had to be careless when she spelled each word and use her worst handwriting.** S: (writes) good/positive; careful; best
14. Writes opposing opinions about a subject using a given set of opposites.	SLP: **Let's prepare for the school writing contest. You will write opposing opinions to debate school rules. Include these opposite words: *fair/unfair*, *early/late*, *pass/fail*.** S1: (writes) A grade of C should be considered passing. S2: (writes) A grade of C is a failing grade.

Synonyms

Yearly Goal: *To develop understanding and spontaneous use of words with similar meanings (synonyms) in listening, speaking, reading, and writing*

CCSS.ELA-LITERACY.L.4.5.C and L.5.5.C

Note: See Appendix B ("Word Lists") for lists to help in planning with these objectives.

Objectives	Examples
1. Chooses the object described by a synonym pair.	SLP: **Look at these objects from our classroom. Point to the one that is skinny and slim.** S: Points to a pencil.
2. Chooses a pair of synonyms to describe an object or picture.	SLP: **Look at this picture and tell me the two synonyms that describe this dog: *animal, flower, pet.*** S: Animal and pet
3. Tells whether two words have the same or opposite meanings.	SLP: **Here are two words from the story we read: *scared, afraid.* Do the words have the same or opposite meanings?** S: Same
4. Given a picture described by two sentences differing in only one word, tells whether the sentences have the same or different meanings.	SLP: **Look at this picture and listen to two sentences about it. Do the sentences have the same or different meanings? Americans won liberty. Americans won freedom.** S: Same
5. Uses a synonym to complete a given sentence.	SLP: **You're learning many synonyms. Use a synonym to make the second sentence mean the same as the first one: The boy was injured. The boy was _____.** S: Hurt
6. Tells which words in a list are synonyms.	SLP: **Listen to these words and tell me which two words mean almost the same: *cheerful, firm, happy, proud.*** S: Cheerful, happy
7. Tells or writes a synonym for each word given.	SLP: **Let's think of some synonyms for your spelling words. What is a synonym for the spelling word *costly*?** S: Expensive
8. Uses a given pair of synonyms in the same sentence.	SLP: **Use these words in the same sentence: *create, make.*** S: When I want to create something, I often make things with clay.

(continues)

Objectives	Examples
9. When given a paragraph, changes its meaning slightly by substituting synonyms for designated words.	SLP: **Change the meaning of this sentence by substituting a synonym: Lincoln wrote the Gettysburg Address.** S: **Lincoln composed the Gettysburg Address.**
10. Explains the difference between the meanings of two sentences that differ only in the synonyms used.	SLP: **Today you'll use your dictionary to compare meanings of these synonyms: *sleep* and *snooze*. Explain why these two sentences with synonyms are not exactly the same: The man sleeps. The man snoozes.** S: **To snooze is to take a short nap, but to sleep is to take either a long nap or a short nap.**

Multiple-Meaning Words

Yearly Goal: *To develop language flexibility through understanding and spontaneous use of multiple-meaning words in listening, speaking, reading, and writing*

CCSS.ELA-LITERACY.L.1.4, L.2.4, L.4.4, L.5.4

Note: See Appendix B ("Word Lists") for lists to help in planning with these objectives.

Objectives	Examples
1. Picks up the correct object or picture when its name is used in a sentence with another meaning.	SLP: **Look at all these objects on the table. Now listen. He can tie his shoe. Pick up another kind of tie.** S: Picks up a necktie.
2. Finds the pictures of a given multiple-meaning word to show its different meanings.	SLP: **On your work sheet, draw a line between the two pictures of *lock*.** S: Draws a line between door lock and lock of hair.
3. Says the word that goes with its two pictured meanings.	SLP: **Look at these pictures. Tell me the word that names both pictures.** S: **Pitcher: baseball pitcher and pitcher of lemonade**
4. Uses the name of a given object or picture correctly in two sentences to show understanding of its different meanings.	SLP: **Look at your pictures and make two sentences to show the meanings of the word *stick*.** S: **This stick came from a tree. I used glue to stick the pictures to the paper.**
5. Names a multiple-meaning word when given two or more definitions.	SLP: **Be a detective and solve the mystery. Look at the three words on the board: *pupil, sharp, cross*. Which word means a part of the eye and also means a school student?** S: **Pupil**

Objectives	Examples
6. Matches a defined multiple-meaning word with its other definition.	SLP: **In the story we finished, the tiger would stalk its prey. Read the sentence on the board that defines another meaning of the word *stalk*.** S: **The sunflower plant has a thick, strong stalk.**
7. Given a list of multiple-meaning words and a list of definitions, matches each word to its appropriate definitions.	SLP: **Let's read this list of words and the other list of definitions. Now tell me two meanings of the word *batter*.** S: **A batter is a person who bats a ball. Batter is also the name for cake or pancake mix.**
8. Tells another definition for a defined multiple-meaning word.	SLP: **Here are pictures of some outdoor scenes. Now we'll work on words with more than one meaning. The word *shade* can mean a color slightly different from another color. Tell another meaning of *shade*.** S: **Shade is a place sheltered from the sun.**
9. Says or writes a multiple-meaning word in sentences to show its different meanings.	SLP: **Let's divide into two teams for this word game. Use the word *mean* in two or more sentences with different meanings.** Team 1: **That angry bull is mean.** Team 2: **I mean what I say.**
10. Tells two or more definitions of each multiple-meaning word.	SLP: **Let's read the words on your list. Choose one of the words from this list and tell two definitions for it: *stir, pound, roll*.** S: ***Stir* can mean to begin to move slightly. It can also mean to move a spoon around in batter to mix it well.**
11. Finds the multiple-meaning words in a paragraph about a selected subject and matches those words to their other definitions.	SLP: **Read this paragraph aloud. Then circle the words that have multiple meanings. Tell another definition for each of those words.** S: **I circled the words *took a plane trip*. *Trip* also means to catch your foot on something and fall.**
12. Explains riddles based on multiple-meaning words.	SLP: **Answer this riddle and tell the class why it's funny: Which object is the king of our classroom?** S: **Ruler. We have a ruler to measure things in our classroom. The joke is funny because *ruler* also means king.**
13. Writes a joke using a multiple-meaning word.	SLP: **With your partner, use a multiple-meaning word to write a joke. Then tell why the joke makes you laugh.** S: (writes) What did the dinosaur say when he ate a clown? That tasted funny. S: **The joke is funny because clowns look funny, and sometimes we say something we ate tasted funny if it has a strange taste.**

Homonyms

Yearly Goal: *To develop understanding and spontaneous use of words that sound the same but have different meanings and spellings (homonyms) in listening, speaking, reading, and writing*

Note: See Appendix B ("Word Lists") for lists to help in planning with these objectives.

Objectives	Examples
1. Points to the picture described by a sentence containing a homonym when looking at pairs of homonym pictures.	SLP: **Look at these pairs of pictures: This is her son. The sun is shining. Point to "The sun is shining."** S: Points to "The sun is shining."
2. Matches a given picture with a picture of its homonym.	SLP: **On this work sheet, draw lines to match pictures of the homonym pairs.** S: Draws a line between pictures of *flower* and *flour*.
3. Uses a pictured homonym correctly in a sentence.	SLP: **See this deer? Use the word *deer* in a sentence.** S: **The deer is in the forest.**
4. Given one homonym in a sentence, creates a new sentence using the other homonym.	SLP: **Your classmate said, "My favorite color is red." Now it's your turn to make a new sentence with the homonym of *red*.** S: **I read a book.**
5. Defines each word in a given homonym pair.	SLP: **What do these words mean: *hair, hare*?** S: **Hair grows on top of your head. A hare is a rabbit.**
6. Indicates whether homonyms are used correctly or incorrectly in written sentences.	SLP: **Read the sentences on this page. Put a plus sign (+) beside the sentence if the correct homonym is used and a minus sign (–) if it is incorrect.** S: (writes) + The sum of two plus two is four.
7. Selects the correct homonym for a given sentence.	SLP: **Look at these sentences that have a choice of two homonyms. Circle the homonym that is correct in this sentence: A *bare/bear* hibernates in the winter.** S: (circles) bear
8. Uses a homonym correctly in a written sentence.	SLP: **Write sentences with these homonyms: *rain/reign*.** S: (writes) The rain is falling. The king had a long reign.
9. Corrects incorrect homonym usage in a story.	SLP: **Rewrite this story by finding and correcting the incorrect homonyms: The wind blue hard. The son was not shining. It started to reign.** S: Corrects homonyms to *blew, sun, rain*.

Objectives	Examples
10. Creates a written paragraph from a list of homonym pairs.	SLP: **Choose three homonym pairs from this grab bag. Now use the homonym pairs you chose to write a paragraph. It's okay if it's a nonsense story.**
11. Uses homonyms correctly in writing a short story.	SLP: **Write a short story using some of these homonyms: *sow/sew, way/weigh, sheer/shear, seem/seam, whole/hole*.**

Word Relationships

Yearly Goal: *To develop the understanding and correct use of word relationships in listening, speaking, reading, and writing*

CCSS.ELA-LITERACY.L.K.5
CCSS.ELA-LITERACY.L.3.1.G
CCSS.ELA-LITERACY.L.8.1.B
CCSS.ELA-LITERACY.W.3.3.C
CCSS.ELA-LITERACY.L.3.6

Note: For more objectives involving word relationships, see Comparatives and Superlatives and Passive Sentences in the Syntax and Morphology unit (Unit 3).

Objectives	Examples
Short-Term Goal: Develops understanding and use of comparative relationships: Damian is taller than Megan.	
1. Answers *yes/no* questions comparing objects.	SLP: **Let's compare some vehicles we've studied. Are buses shorter than cars?** S: **No**
2. Answers true or false questions comparing objects.	SLP: **Let's look at the items your classmates brought to show-and-tell. True or false? Bart's drum is louder than Emma's book.** S: **True**
3. Points to the picture that shows the meaning of a comparative relationship given in a sentence.	SLP: **Look at these pictures on the bulletin board. Find this picture: The hot-air balloon is flying higher than the airplane.**
4. Orally completes sentences comparing objects.	SLP: **Let's take a walk around the school. Now finish my sentence: The trees are taller than the _____.** S: **Bushes**
5. Writes a description of a picture using a comparative word relationship.	SLP: **Write a comparative sentence about this picture.** S: (writes) The giraffe is taller than the llama.

(continues)

Objectives	Examples
Short-Term Goal: Develops understanding and use of passive relationships: The car was driven by Russ.	
6. Judges the meaning of a pair of passive and declarative sentences as the same or different.	SLP: **Think about our science lesson. Is the meaning of these two sentences the same or different? The lima beans were planted by the class. The class planted the lima beans.** S: **Same**
7. Answers questions about passive sentences.	SLP: **We are going to talk about what just happened. The pencil was sharpened by Pam. Who sharpened the pencil?** S: **Pam**
8. Points to the picture that shows the meaning of a passive relationship within a sentence.	SLP: **Look at the pictures on this work sheet and point to this one: The boy was chased by the dog.**
9. Sequences a spoken scrambled sentence about a picture.	SLP: **Listen to these words from our social studies lesson and make a new sentence from them: *was written by Francis Scott Key the song*.** S: **The song was written by Francis Scott Key.**
10. Writes, reads, and acts out a sentence that contains a passive word relationship.	SLP: **Read this passive sentence that David wrote and then act it out.** S: (reads and acts out) **The boy is stung by a bee.**
Short-Term Goal: Develops understanding and use of time–sequence relationships: February comes before March.	
11. Points to the place on a calendar requested in a time–sequence relationship.	SLP: **It's Calendar Time! Point to the day that comes after Monday.** S: Points to *Tuesday*.
12. Answers true-or-false questions about pictured time–sequence relationships.	SLP: **Use these pictures about time to help you answer my questions. Is this true or false? Fall comes after winter.** S: **False**
13. Completes sentences about pictures using time–sequence relationships.	SLP: **Here is a calendar about our school activities. Complete my sentence. We'll go to the symphony in March and have Field Day one month later. We'll have Field Day in _____.** S: **April**
14. Writes a sentence to describe a picture using a time–sequence relationship.	SLP: **Look at this calendar with your classmates' birthdays. Write a time–sequence sentence about two of your classmates' birthdays.** S: (writes) Raul's birthday is two weeks before Maria's.
Short-Term Goal: Develops understanding and use of familial relationships: My uncle is my dad's brother.	
15. Answers questions about people in immediate familial relationships.	SLP: **Let's make a poster showing the people in your immediate family. Point to your father's son.**

Objectives	Examples
16. Answers true-or-false questions about familial relationships shown in pictures.	SLP: **Look at this family picture you brought today and answer some questions. Is this true or false? Your father's brother is your brother.** S: **False**
17. Completes sentences using familial relationships.	SLP: **Complete this sentence. Albert's father's father is Albert's _____.** S: **Grandfather**
18. Writes sentences using familial relationships for everyone who lives in his or her house.	SLP: **Write some sentences to tell how everyone who lives in your house is related.** S: (writes) My father is married to my mother. My mother's mother is my grandmother. My parents' son is my brother.

Verbal Analogies

Yearly Goal: *To improve semantic abilities and thinking skills through understanding and spontaneous use of analogies in listening, speaking, reading, and writing*

CCSS.ELA-LITERACY.L.7.5.B

Teaching Note: Introduce analogies in active, affirmative, declarative sentences. For example, "A dog barks, but a cat meows." Gradually move to the formal construction "_____ is to _____ as _____ is to _____." The relative order of difficulty for the various types of verbal analogies is presented in this section.

Note: See Appendix B ("Word Lists") for examples of different types of verbal analogies.

Objectives	Examples
1. Uses one word to complete a simple analogy.	SLP: **Finish this: A dog has a nose. An elephant has a _____.** S: **Trunk**
2. Identifies the critical words in a verbal analogy represented with objects.	SLP: **Look at these stuffed animals of a dog and a duck. A dog has fur, and a duck has feathers. Which word tells what covers a dog? Which word tells what covers a duck?** S: **Fur; feathers**
3. Judges the consistency of the expressed relationship within a verbal analogy represented with pictures.	SLP: **Look at these pictures from our jungle animal story. Is this analogy right or wrong? A leopard has spots, but a zebra has stripes.** S: **Right**
4. Chooses the pictured word that correctly completes a verbal analogy.	SLP: **Think about our lesson on body parts, and choose the correct word: Feet have toes like hands have *skin* or *fingers*.** S: **Fingers**

(continues)

Objectives	Examples
5. Tells the answer to a verbal analogy.	SLP: **Finish this analogy: Mother is to daughter as father is to _____.** S: **Son**
6. Writes an answer to a written analogy.	SLP: **On this work sheet, write the correct answer to this analogy: Chef is to cook as physician is to _____.** S: (writes) doctor
7. Creates analogies.	SLP: **Use these words to create an analogy: *continent, nation.*** S: **Continent is to Australia as nation is to Canada.**

Figurative Language

Yearly Goal: *To develop vocabulary and meaning by increasing understanding and spontaneous use of figurative language: idioms, similes, metaphors, and proverbs*

CCSS.ELA-LITERACY.L.4.5
CCSS.ELA-LITERACY.L.3.5.A–L.5.5.A
CCSS.ELA-LITERACY.L.4.5.B and L.5.5.B

Note: Examples of figurative language are in Appendix B.

Objectives	Examples
1. Chooses the correct meaning of a spoken figurative expression when its literal and figurative meanings are acted out.	SLP: **Hannah and Ava acted out the figurative and literal meanings of "Aaron was an eager beaver." Which showed the correct meaning?** S: The correct meaning was when they acted like they just couldn't wait to start the trip. That was the figurative meaning.
2. Selects the picture that shows the intended meaning of a spoken figurative expression.	SLP: **Look at these pictures. Describe the one that shows newborn seals as hungry as bears.** S: **It's the picture of the seals eating.**
3. Answers true-or-false questions about literal and figurative sentences.	SLP: **True or false? If I say "Jason's dog was happy as a clam," I think his dog is a clam.** S: **False**
4. Finds the words in a figurative statement that create an image.	SLP: **Pull a figurative sentence from these cards. Which words create an image rather than describe a fact? The moon was as round as a silver dollar.** S: **As round as a silver dollar**
5. Matches figurative spoken sentences with their meanings.	SLP: **Figurative expressions help us imagine what was described. What does it mean to say "the tiger had emerald eyes"?** S: **They were shiny green like emeralds.**

Objectives	Examples
6. Identifies figurative language in a paragraph read aloud.	SLP: **Find the figurative sentence in this paragraph: Children love the reading rug. It's special. Walking on the rug is like walking on air.** S: Walking on the rug is like walking on air.
7. Tells why a figurative expression in a paragraph or story would be absurd if interpreted literally.	SLP: **Figurative language sounds absurd if you think about it literally. Why is the literal meaning of "catch a cold" absurd?** S: You can't run after a bad cold. It's an illness.
8. Explains the abstract meanings of idioms, metaphors, similes, or proverbs within context.	SLP: **Explain to the class what this sentence means: John said, "I can't eat this soup. It's hot as fire!"** S: His soup is too hot to eat right away.
9. Creates original similes and metaphors by changing existing ones used in a sentence or paragraph.	SLP: **Create a new figurative expression for this expression: The sisters were like two peas in a pod.** S: The sisters were like two eggs in a nest.
10. Matches a proverb to a story.	SLP: **Listen carefully. I want you to choose the proverb that matches this fable: A fox sneered at a lioness, "You never give birth to more than one cub, but I can birth six baby foxes." "Yes, only one," the lioness replied, "but it's a lion." Choose the better proverb: (1) It's quality not quantity that counts. (2) Honesty is the best policy.** S: It is quality not quantity that counts.
11. Gives a generalized moral ending to a short story or fable by creating a proverb to summarize its abstract meaning.	SLP: **In this story, a boy put off his work and then missed the movie. Let's create a proverb.** S: Work done first leaves time for play.

Inferences, Predictions, and Outcomes

Yearly Goal: *To perceive, explain, or use hidden, unstated verbal meanings and to grasp their implications, absurdities, inferences, outcomes, and predictions*

CCSS.ELA-LITERACY.CCRA.R.1
CCSS.ELA-LITERACY.RL.4.1

Objectives	Examples
Short-Term Goal: Understands and uses inconsistencies and absurdities	
1. Detects inconsistencies or absurdities in pictures or in a role play.	SLP: **Here are some silly pictures. Explain what's absurd in them. A boy is talking into a pencil as if it's a telephone.** S: You write with a pencil.

(continues)

Objectives	Examples
2. Detects inconsistencies or absurdities in a pictured scene.	SLP: **Look at this picture of horses at a rodeo. What's wrong here?** S: **Horses don't have horns; cows do.**
3. Explains inconsistencies or absurdities in a pictured scene.	SLP: **This picture doesn't make sense. Why?** S: **It shows penguins in a desert with camels. Penguins live in cold places, not deserts.**
4. Corrects inconsistencies or absurdities in verbal materials of increasing length and complexity (sentences, paragraphs, stories, recorded dialogues).	SLP: **Correct the word in this sentence that doesn't make sense: Three hundred miles is a short distance.** S: **Three hundred miles is a long distance.**
5. Explains inconsistencies in verbal materials of increasing length and complexity (sentences, paragraphs, stories, recorded dialogues).	SLP: **Listen. Ryan was scared when he saw the thunder in the mountains. Explain what was wrong in that sentence.** S: **You hear thunder. You don't see it.**
Short-Term Goal: Predicts future outcomes	
6. Predicts future outcomes of pictured situations by selecting what will happen next from among several outcomes.	SLP: **Let's make predictions about these picture scenes. Allison is turning in her homework, and the teacher is smiling. Will Allison be punished, or will she get a sticker?** S: **She'll get a sticker.**
7. Predicts future outcomes of pictured situations.	SLP: **In this picture, storm clouds are gathering over the lake. What might happen next?** S: **There might be thunder, lightning, and rain.**
8. Predicts what a story or book will be about based on its title and several pictures.	SLP: **Look at the title and cover of the book *Bringing the Rain to Kapiti Plain*. Predict what you think it will be about.** S: **It shows a picture of a desert that needs rain. Maybe the people will do something to get it to rain.**
9. Predicts an appropriate ending to a story or situation.	SLP: **Now you've heard most of the story about the drought on Kapiti Plain. How do you think the story will end?** S: **The rain will finally come.**
Short-Term Goal: Identifies possible causes	
10. Identifies several possible causes of pictured predicaments or situations.	SLP: **Let's talk about possible causes or reasons things happened. In this picture, a plant is wilted. What could have caused this?** S: **The plant got too much water. It didn't get enough water. It got a plant disease.**

Objectives	Examples
12. Identifies several possible causes of stated predicaments or situations.	SLP: **In the book *Miss Nelson Is Missing*, the teacher didn't come to teach her class today. Tell several causes.** S: **Perhaps she got sick. A family member had an accident. Her car broke down.**
Short-Term Goal: Understands and explains inferences	
13. Makes appropriate inferences about a pictured situation based on available information or evidence.	SLP: **In this picture we see Joshua walking home from school. He sees a deliveryman leaving a package on his front porch. We know that Josh ordered a new computer game. How do you think he feels?** S: **He's excited. He thinks it might be his game.**
14. Explains appropriate inferences about stated situations based on available information or evidence.	SLP: **Listen and explain how Mother feels. Mother surveyed the messy kitchen, put her hands on her hips, and demanded of the children, "What's going on here?"** S: **She feels angry.**
Short-Term Goal: Interprets and explains facts or opinions	
15. Identifies statements in advertisements as facts or opinions.	SLP: **We're learning how to interpret facts and opinions, and we watched a video of an advertisement. Is this statement a fact or an opinion? You will be more beautiful if you use Breath Fresh.** S: **Opinion**
16. Writes a fact statement and an opinion statement for a product.	SLP: **Today our grab bag has pictures of products we might buy. Pull out a picture. Then write two statements about your product. One will be a fact, and one will be an opinion.** S: (writes) Fact: Sunrise Breakfast Cereal is crunchy. Opinion: You will feel great if you start each morning with a bowl of this cereal.
Short-Term Goal: Interprets and explains changes in meaning implied by intonation and juncture	
17. Interprets changes in meaning signaled by intonation, pitch, intensity, duration, rate, and juncture.	SLP: **We can get clues about what someone means by the emphasis on his or her words. Listen to Jonathan say each sentence in different ways. Raise your hand when the sentence means that it's only the paper that he wants.** ***Give* the paper to me.** **Give the paper to *me*.** **Give the *paper* to me.** S: Raises hand on last sentence.

(continues)

Objectives	Examples
18. Explains meaning changes in sentence pairs signaled by subtle changes in juncture.	SLP: **Listen for tiny pauses that change the meanings of words:** **He is a grand father.** **He is a grandfather.** **Draw a picture of the last one I said.** S: Draws a picture of an older man who could be a grandfather.
19. Explains differences between surface messages and underlying messages in sentences.	SLP: **Implied meaning gives additional information to actual words in a sentence. Tell me the surface meaning and then the implied meaning of this sentence: The man wearing the dirty shirt spoke at the meeting.** S: **Surface: The speaker wore a dirty shirt. Implied: Don't take his message seriously.**
20. Writes a paragraph or story that contains an unstated theme, inference, or underlying message.	SLP: **Write a paragraph that describes a character's actions without stating the character's feelings. We will guess the character's feelings.** S: (writes) George didn't have any trouble going to sleep, but morning came too soon. He groaned. He couldn't believe his body could hurt more than it had the day before. The only thing that got him out of bed was the first light of morning. The blistering sun would rise soon.

Unit 3

Syntax and Morphology

- Negatives
- Asking *Wh-* Questions
- Asking *Yes/No* Questions
- Pronouns
- Plural Nouns
- Copular (Linking) and Auxiliary (Helping) Verbs
- Possessive Nouns
- Comparatives and Superlatives
- Past Tense Verbs
- Third Person Verbs
- Infinitives
- Future Tense Verbs
- Articles
- Conjunctions and Transition Words
- Modal Auxiliaries
- Complex Sentences
- Passive Sentences

Conveying ideas through speech or writing demands knowledge of word- and sentence-formation rules. These rules include those for morphemes and syntax. A *morpheme* is a meaningful unit of language, and morphology is the set of rules that govern the use of morphemes. A morpheme is the smallest grammatical unit that is indivisible without violating the meaning or producing meaningless units (Owens, 2016). The rules for forming plurals, possessives, verb tenses, and other meaningful units of language are morphological rules. There are also rules for putting those words together into sentences. *Syntax* refers to those rules. These rules specify word, phrase, and clause order; sentence organization; and the relationships among words, word classes, and other sentence elements. Syntax specifies which word combinations are acceptable, or grammatical, and which are not (Owens, 2016). Passive sentences, complex sentences, and interrogatives are all structured according to the syntactical rules of the English language. The ability to accurately interpret the structural and semantic aspects of language is dependent on the knowledge of these rules.

Syntax and morphology play a crucial part in both spoken and written language. In spoken language, the speaker must be able to use the structure, and the listener must know the rules and be able to understand them for communication to take place. The same is true in written language. The writer and the reader must follow morphological and syntactical rules if the correct message is to be conveyed. The formulation and production of oral and written language affects all learning and human interactions. A good understanding of the rules for syntax and morphology is essential to this process.

The objectives in this unit provide help in planning lessons that facilitate the development of syntax and morphology in students whose assessments have shown deficits in these areas. These objectives can be used in association with a variety of language programs. Conversational approaches that use natural situations to stimulate interactions and the language arts curriculum of the classroom are especially suitable. Owens (2010) pointed out that making syntactic training as conversational as possible is important so that the student can learn to use the rules in context. Contextual practice of utterances strengthens the relationships across linguistic units.

Each section in this unit begins with a receptive task and, when appropriate, progresses from the imitated one-word level to phrases, sentences, conversation, and writing. In many cases, several sections could be taught together to reinforce each other. For example, the sections Pronouns (pp. 72–76) and Copular (Linking) and Auxiliary (Helping) Verbs (pp. 78–80) could be used together for the child to form sentences such as "She is pretty" and "They are swimming." A standardized language test or a complete language sample analysis are excellent measures for determining which areas and which levels of syntax and morphology are appropriate targets.

Appendix B contains the following materials that may be helpful when planning intervention using the objectives in this unit:

- Pronouns
- Plurals: Regular and Irregular
- Irregular Past Tense Verbs
- Conjunctions
- Transition Words

Appendix D contains information on sentence types.

Negatives

Yearly Goal: *To develop the understanding and correct use of negatives when listening, speaking, reading, and writing*

CCSS.ELA-LITERACY.L.K.4.B
CCSS.ELA-LITERACY.L.3.4.B
CCSS.ELA-LITERACY.L.5.2.C

Objectives	Examples
1. Answers *no* to "Is this a _____?" when shown an incorrectly named object.	SLP: **Look at the toy I'm playing with. Is it a block?** S: **No. It's a car.**
2. Answers *no* when asked about things not liked or needed.	SLP: **Do you need help?** S: **No.**
3. Chooses objects or pictures described with a phrase or sentence containing the word *not*.	SLP: **Look at the toys on the shelf. Touch a toy that is not a car. Bring me a block that is not blue.**
4. Uses *not* in phrases or sentences to describe pictures of opposites.	SLP: **Tell me about these pictures of opposites. Use the word *not*.** S: **Happy baby. Not happy. The elephant is big. The mouse is not big.**
5. Uses *not* in phrases or sentences to describe activities or surroundings.	SLP: **Use the word *not* to tell about things that you see happening in the classroom.** S: **Not quiet. Scott is not reading.**
6. Uses *don't*, *can't*, *won't*, *wouldn't*, or *shouldn't* to answer a question.	SLP: **Answer my questions about what is happening on the playground. Can he run faster than you?** S: **No, he can't.** SLP: **Do you want to go inside now?** S: **No, I don't.**
7. Uses negatives to ask questions.	SLP: **Use some words that mean no to ask your friend questions about playing football.** S: **Why don't you play football? Why won't you try out for the team? Why not?**
8. Uses *isn't* or *aren't* to describe a picture.	SLP: **Look at these pictures from our food lesson. What food am I talking about? It isn't sweet.** S: **A lemon isn't sweet.**
9. Uses *isn't* or *doesn't* to tell about people or objects.	SLP: **Use the words *isn't* or *doesn't* to tell about who you see as we walk around in the school.** S: **Mrs. Maxwell doesn't teach music. Penny isn't the principal.**
10. Uses negatives to describe differences.	SLP: **Look at these books we got from the library. How are these two books different?** S: **The red book isn't as funny as the blue book.**

(continues)

Objectives	Examples
11. Points to the correct pictures when hearing words with prefixes *un-*, *non-*, *dis-*.	SLP: **Look at these opposite pictures. Show me *unhappy*.**
12. Uses the prefixes *un-*, *non-*, *dis-* to complete a sentence.	SLP: **Look at these pictures and complete my sentence. This boy is happy. This girl is _____.** S: **unhappy**
13. Uses *wouldn't* or *shouldn't* to explain the solution to a problem.	SLP: **Use the words *wouldn't* or *shouldn't* to answer my question. How should students not act in the hallway?** S: **They shouldn't run.**
14. Uses negatives to state an opinion.	SLP: **Use some words that mean *no* to talk about which snack food we need.** S: **I don't think we should have popcorn. I can't eat peanuts.**
15. Uses negatives in conversation.	SLP: **During our group discussion, be sure to use words that mean *no* correctly while we talk about animals that do and do not live in the ocean.** S: **Elephants don't live in the ocean.**
16. Uses negatives in written answers to questions.	SLP: **Think about the video we just watched. Why didn't the flower grow?** S: (writes) They didn't water it.
17. Uses a comma to set off the words *yes* and *no* in a written answer.	SLP: **Write your answer to my questions.** S: (writes) No, I can't come. Yes, that's my name.
18. Uses negatives to write a paragraph that retells a favorite story.	SLP: **You just told me your favorite story. Now write a paragraph about it and try to use some of the words that mean *not*. What are some words you could use in your paragraph?** S: **no, not, couldn't, don't, can't** Writes a paragraph using negative words.
19. Uses negatives in all writing.	SLP: **Be sure to use negatives correctly in today's writing lesson.**

Asking *Wh-* Questions

Yearly Goal: *To develop the understanding and correct use of* wh- *questions in speaking, reading, and writing*

CCSS.ELA-LITERACY.RL.K.1–R.L.3.1
CCSS.ELA-LITERACY.RL.K.4
CCSS.ELA-LITERACY.RI.3.1
CCSS.ELA-LITERACY.SL.K.2
CCSS.ELA-LITERACY.SL.K.3 and SL.2.3
CCSS.ELA-LITERACY.L.K.1.D

Objectives	Examples
1. Imitates the SLP or says single words with a rising intonation that indicate *wh-* questions.	SLP: **Mommy?** S: **Mommy?** for Where's Mommy?
2. Imitates the SLP or says two-word questions beginning with *what* or *who*.	SLP: **Look at our book. Say this: Who eat? What that?**
3. Imitates the SLP or says the following where questions: *where* + noun, *where* + verb, or *where* + noun + verb.	SLP: **Let's play and I will hide some toys. Say this: Where truck? Where swim? Where baby sleep?**
4. Asks *what* questions to learn the meaning of a new word heard in conversation or in a text.	SLP: **Ask me a question if you don't know a word from our story.** S: **What's a caterpillar?**
5. Asks structured *who* + *is* or *what* + *is* questions about a picture.	SLP: **Look at this picture and ask questions that begin with *Who is* or *What is*.** S: **Who is sleeping? What is flying?**
6. Asks structured *where* + *is* questions about hidden objects or pictures.	SLP: **I'm going to hide an object in the room. To find it, ask a question that starts with *Where is*.** S: **Where is the pencil?**
7. Asks structured *how* and *why* questions while participating in an activity.	SLP: **To find out more about our experiment, ask some questions that begin with *How* or *Why*.** S: **How did the water turn purple? Why did we use food coloring?**
8. Asks structured *when* questions about an activity.	SLP: **To find out about our daily routine, ask some questions that begin with *When*.** S: **When does school start? When can we go outside?**
9. Completes *wh-* questions in a spoken cloze task.	SLP: **Think about the book we just read and finish this question. Whales are mammals that live in the ocean. What _____?** S: **are whales?** SLP: **Where _____?** S: **do whales live?**

(continues)

Objectives	Examples
10. Asks *wh-* questions that are requested.	SLP: **Ask a *where* question about this picture of the library.** S: **Where are the books about sports?**
11. Rewords a stated *wh-* question.	SLP: **Ask this question another way: What person is the leader today?** S: **Who is the leader today?**
12. Asks *wh-* questions about pictures.	SLP: **Ask a *wh-* question about this picture of different animals.** S: **Which of these animals is the fastest?**
13. Asks a peer *wh-* questions about a reading assignment.	SLP: **Take turns asking your partner *wh-* questions about the story you just read.**
14. Uses *wh-* questions to ask for information, permission, clarification, and reasons.	SLP: **What question could you ask to find out more information about a school assignment?** S: **When is it due?**
15. Asks *wh-* questions while role playing an interview.	SLP: **Ask *wh-* questions as you interview Paul Revere after his midnight ride.** S: **What was the name of your horse? When did you start your ride?**
16. Asks *wh-* questions about key details in a text that is read or that is presented orally.	SLP: **Ask *wh-* questions for your classmates to answer about the key details of this story.** S: **Who is the main character? Where is the setting? When did this story take place?**
17. Writes a *wh-* question to get requested information.	SLP: **Write a *wh-* question on the board to find out the favorite snack of sixth graders.** S: (writes) What do sixth graders like best for snacks?
18. Writes *wh-* questions about a paragraph for a peer to answer.	SLP: **Let's practice for the quiz. Write three *wh-* questions for your partner to answer.**

Asking *Yes/No* Questions

Yearly Goal: *To use a variety of* yes/no *questions correctly when speaking, reading, and writing*

CCSS.ELA-LITERACY.RL.K.1 and RL.1.1
CCSS.ELA-LITERACY.RL.K.4
CCSS.ELA-LITERACY.RI.1.4
CCSS.ELA-LITERACY.SL.K.2 and SL.1.2
CCSS.ELA-LITERACY.SL.K.3 and SL.1.3
CCSS.ELA-LITERACY.SL.1.1.C

Objectives	Examples
1. Produces or imitates the SLP's rising intonation in single words to indicate *yes/no* questions.	SLP: **Listen to me ask you a question. Ball? More?** (with rising intonation) **Now you ask me.** S: Imitates or asks single word *yes/no* questions.
2. Imitates the SLP as she says two-word phrases with rising intonation to ask *yes/no* questions.	SLP: **Say what I say when I ask you some questions. Go outside? Coat on?** (with rising intonation) S: Imitates or asks two-word *yes/no* questions.
3. Imitates *yes/no* questions about objects or situations.	SLP: **See Danny. Danny is sitting. Let's ask a question. "Is Danny sitting?" Now you ask the question.** S: **Is Danny sitting?**
4. Creates a *yes/no* question about a picture from the declarative sentence and the first word of the question.	SLP: **The girl is painting. Make this sentence into a question. Begin with *is*.** S: **Is the girl painting?**
5. Thinks of all of the words that can be used to begin *yes/no* questions.	SLP: **Think of all of the words that can be used to begin *yes/no* questions. I will write them on the board as you think of them.** S: ***is, are, was, were, has, have, had, does, do, did, can, may, might, could, should, would, will***
6. Changes a given *yes/no* question about a picture into another *yes/no* question.	SLP: **Do you think he will win the race? Now ask this question in a different way.** S: **Can he win the race?**
7. Asks *yes/no* questions to seek help, to gain information, to clarify, and to learn the meaning of unknown words.	SLP: **Where does Allison want to go on vacation? Ask her some *yes/no* questions to find out.** S: **Will you ride on an airplane? Is it cold there? Can you play in the snow? Will you wear a coat?**
8. Asks *yes/no* questions about information read aloud.	SLP: **Ask *yes/no* questions to find out more about the story we just read.** S: **Did the firemen come? Was the dog okay?**

(continues)

Objectives	Examples
9. Asks *yes/no* questions about key details in a text.	SLP: **Ask *yes/no* questions for your classmates to answer about the key details of this story.** S: **Is the main character a boy? Does he live in the city?**
10. Asks *yes/no* questions in structured conversation.	SLP: **In your small group, ask each other *yes/no* questions about the lesson to help study for your test.** S: **Was George Washington the first U.S. president?**
11. Writes a *yes/no* question when given a question word.	SLP: **Write a question about Betsy Ross that begins with the word *does*.** S: (writes) Does the flag today look the same as the one Betsy Ross made?
12. Writes *yes/no* questions about a picture.	SLP: **Write *yes/no* questions about these pictures from the story you just heard.** S: (writes) Do insects have eight legs?
13. Writes *yes/no* questions about a story or event.	SLP: **I want you and your partner to write five *yes/no* questions about the article you read. Then write answers to each other's questions.**

Pronouns

Yearly Goal: *To develop understanding and correct use of pronouns when listening, speaking, reading, and writing*

CCSS.ELA-LITERACY.RF.K.3.C
CCSS.ELA-LITERACY.L.1.1.D
CCSS.ELA-LITERACY.L.2.1.C
CCSS.ELA-LITERACY.L.4.1.A
CCSS.ELA-LITERACY.L.6.1.A–L.6.1.D

Note: Refer to Appendix B ("Word Lists") for a list of the most common pronouns.

Objectives	Examples
Short-Term Goal: Understands and uses personal subject pronouns *I, you, he, she, it, we, they*	
1. Given the single-word pronoun *he*, *she*, or *they*, points to the correct picture.	SLP: **Look at these pictures. Point to *he*. Point to *she*. Point to *they*.** S: Points to a boy, a girl, and a group of people.
2. Chooses the action or picture described using personal subject pronouns.	SLP: **Look at our library book and show me, "She is climbing." Show me, "They are playing soccer."**

Objectives	Examples
3. Discriminates between correct and incorrect personal subject pronouns in spoken sentences.	SLP: **Show me thumbs-up if this sounds right and thumbs-down if this sounds wrong. Me run fast. He has a book. Them are singing.** S: thumbs-down, thumbs-up, thumbs-down
4. Imitates the SLP using the personal subject pronouns *I*, *he*, *she*, *you*, *it*, and *they* in short sentences.	SLP: **Let's talk about your friends on the playground. Say what I say: I see. He can run. She kicks. They play.**
5. Says personal subject pronouns in phrases or sentences to describe pictures.	SLP: **Look at these pictures and answer my questions. What is the man doing in this picture?** S: **He is building a house.**
6. Given a spoken sentence, replaces proper nouns with pronouns.	SLP: **Change this sentence by using a pronoun: John is sick today.** S: **He is sick today.**
7. Corrects pronouns used incorrectly in spoken sentences.	SLP: **Make my sentence correct: "John is a farmer. Him grows food for us to eat."** S: **He grows food for us to eat.**
Short-Term Goal: Understands and uses the personal object pronouns *me, you, him, her, it, us, you, them*	
8. Chooses the action or picture described with personal object pronouns.	SLP: **Look at this picture scene and point to what I am talking about. Shirley gave the ball to him. The trophy goes to them.**
9. Discriminates between correct and incorrect use of object pronouns heard in sentences.	SLP: **Hold up the green card if my sentence is correct and the red card if it is wrong. I will call she. Let's save some dessert for they. I want to play with him.** S: Holds up red card, red card, green card.
10. Given a spoken sentence, replaces proper names with correct subject pronouns.	SLP: **Circle the correct pronoun to use in this sentence: This book belongs to Amy.** S: (circles) her
11. Uses personal subject pronouns correctly in spoken sentences.	SLP: **Take a card from the bag. Use this word in a sentence.** S: Chooses the word *me*. Says, **Give it to me.**
Short-Term Goal: Understands and uses the possessive pronouns *my, mine, your, yours, his, its, her, hers, they, theirs, our, ours*	
12. Chooses correct pictures that are described with possessive pronouns.	SLP: **Bring me the picture I am talking about. The car is his. Today is her birthday. Their team is the winner.**
13. Discriminates between correct and incorrect use of personal pronouns in sentences.	SLP: **Color the happy face if what I say is correct and the sad face if it is wrong. This is she coat. My friend is happy. He mom is here.** S: Colors the sad face, happy face, sad face.

(continues)

Objectives	Examples
14. Completes a sentence with the correct personal pronoun.	SLP: **Finish my sentence with the correct pronoun: The fire truck is_____. The hammer is _____.** S: **theirs, his**
15. Uses personal pronouns in short sentences.	SLP: **Use the correct pronoun to tell whose turn it is while we play this board game.** S: **It's my turn. It's his/her turn. It's your turn. The next turn is his/hers.**
Short-Term Goal: Understands and uses indefinite pronouns, such as *all, anyone, everybody, few, many, someone*	
16. Chooses pictures that are described with indefinite pronouns.	SLP: **Look at my picture pairs about a birthday party. Point to the picture I am describing. All the guests are wearing party hats. A few of the children are eating. No one is crying. Several of the children are standing up.**
17. When given an indefinite pronoun, uses it correctly in a sentence.	SLP: **Hit one of the cards on the wall with the beanbag. Now use that word in a sentence.** S: Hits *anyone*. Says, **Does anyone know the answer?**
18. Uses indefinite pronouns in sentences.	SLP: **Look at this list of indefinite pronouns on the board: *everyone, both, many*. Use them to tell about what is happening in our room.** S: **Everyone is sitting at a desk. Both of my friends are here. Many of them have a pencil.**
Short-Term Goal: Understands and uses the reflexive pronouns *myself, yourself, himself, herself, itself, ourselves, yourselves, themselves*	
19. Chooses pictures that are described with reflexive pronouns.	SLP: **Circle the picture I am talking about. She painted the picture by herself. The chef burned himself yesterday. Everyone is eating.**
20. Completes a sentence with the correct relative pronoun.	SLP: **Finish my sentence: I don't want you to hear the story from Dan; I want to tell you the story _____. The girls walked home by _____. He built the model by _____.** S: **Myself, themselves, himself**
21. When given a reflexive pronoun, uses it correctly in a sentence.	SLP: **Before you take a turn in this board game, use the reflexive pronoun I say: *myself, herself*.** S: **I don't want my brother to read it, I want to read it myself. My sister can ride a bike by herself.**

Objectives	Examples
Short-Term Goal: Understands and uses the relative pronouns *this, these, that, those*	
22. Chooses pictures that are described with relative pronouns.	SLP: **Here are sets of picture pairs. Point to the picture I am talking about. Where is the dog that was lost? These are my favorite pencils. Where are those maps you bought? Is this what you are looking for?**
23. Completes a sentence with the correct relative pronoun.	SLP: **Read this list of pronouns. Choose a relative pronoun to complete each sentence. Let's don't light that tall candle; Let's light _____ short candle. Yesterday I wore those brown shoes, but today I am wearing _____ red ones. This puppy is so cute; so is _____ one.** S: **This, these, that**
23. When given a relative pronoun, uses it correctly in a sentence.	SLP: **Use *this, these, that,* or *those* to talk about the softball game.** S: **Sandra hit that fly ball hard. Those new bats were great. I hope these teams play again.**
Short-Term Goal: Understands and uses all forms of pronouns	
24. Reads a list of sight words that include common pronouns.	SLP: **Read these words aloud as quickly as you can.**
25. Understands and corrects pronouns with unclear or ambiguous antecedents.	SLP: **Change my sentences to make them more clear: (1) Allison told Sherrie to come at 3:00, but she was late. (2) The paint can was on the ladder when it fell.** S: **(1) Allison told Sherrie to come at 3:00, but Sherrie was late. (2) When the ladder fell, the paint can was on it.**
26. Uses pronouns to retell short stories.	SLP: **Use pronouns to summarize the information we learned.** S: **We talked about the United States flag. It is red, white, and blue. That is the flag that flies at our school.**
27. Given written sentences, corrects pronoun usage.	SLP: **Correct the pronoun used incorrectly in this sentence: Them went to battle in 1836.** S: (writes) They went to battle in 1836.
28. Rewrites a paragraph replacing proper nouns with pronouns.	SLP: **Rewrite this article, replacing proper nouns with pronouns: Angela Blackstone is a local attorney. The office on the top floor belongs to Angela. You can read more about Angela on her website.** S: (writes) She is a local attorney. The office on the top floor belongs to her. You can read more about her on her website.

(continues)

Objectives	Examples
29. Uses pronouns to write about a previous event.	SLP: **Use pronouns to write a paragraph to summarize what we did in science class.** S: (writes) Yesterday we read about insects. There are thousands of them. They are amazing animals.
30. Uses pronouns to write short stories.	SLP: **Use some pronouns to write a short story about an expedition in space travel.** S: (writes) It is the year 2419. We are exploring our universe. (and so on)

Plural Nouns

Yearly Goal: *To develop the understanding and correct use of plural nouns when listening, speaking, reading, and writing*

CCSS.ELA-LITERACY.L.K.1.C
CCSS.ELA-LITERACY.L.1.1.C
CCSS.ELA-LITERACY.L.2.1.B and L.3.1.B
CCSS.ELA-LITERACY.L.3.1.B

Note: Please refer to Appendix B ("Word Lists") for a list of the most common regular and irregular plurals.

Objectives	Examples
Short-Term Goal: Understands and uses singular or regular plural nouns	
1. Points to singular or regular plural objects as they are named.	SLP: **I have hidden some things around the room. Do what I say. Go find a pencil. Find the cups. Bring me the books.** S: Follows directions correctly, bringing one or more objects as requested.
2. Imitates the SLP's model as singular or regular plural objects are labeled.	SLP: **This is a book. Say *book*. These are two books. Say *books*.** S: **Says *book* then *books*.**
3. Indicates when regular plural nouns are spoken.	SLP: **Show me thumbs up when I say a word that means more than one: *dog, cats*.**
4. Given pictures to choose from, points to singular or regular plural nouns named.	SLP: **Look at these pictures. Show me the ball. Point to all the balloons.** S: Points to a picture of a ball, then points to a picture of balloons.
5. Follows spoken directions that require understanding of singular or regular plural concepts.	SLP: **Look at the pictures on this work sheet. Draw a circle around the bike. Draw a box around the bikes.**
6. Says the regular plural or singular form of pictured nouns.	SLP: **Let's look out the window at the playground. What do you see?** S: **I see monkey bars, a girl, swings.**

Objectives	Examples
Short-Term Goal: Uses singular and plural nouns with matching verbs in basic sentences: "He hops." "We hop."	
7. Points to the singular or plural action when described in a two-word sentence.	SLP: **Watch your classmates do some actions. Point to "He hops." Point to "They hop."**
8. Points to the correct singular or plural picture as described in a two-word sentence.	SLP: **Look at all of these action pictures. Put a token on "She sleeps." Put a token on "They sleep."**
9. Imitates the SLP's models of two-word singular and plural sentences.	SLP: **Look at the pictures in our book. These children are running. Say "They run." The puppy is barking. Say "Puppy barks."**
10. Follows directions that contain singular and plural nouns with matching verbs.	SLP: **Let's play with these stuffed animals. Show me "Bear jumps." Now show me "Dogs run."** S: Makes the toy bear jump and the toy dog run.
11. Says the correct two-word sentences with singular and plural nouns and matching verbs.	SLP: **Look at these pictures. What does he do?** S: **He slides.**
Short-Term Goal: Understands and uses singular or irregular plural nouns	
12. Points to singular or irregular plural objects and pictures as they are named.	SLP: **Follow my directions on this work sheet. Circle the feet. Put an X on the goose.**
13. Imitates the SLP's model as singular or irregular plural objects and pictures are labeled.	SLP: **Let's see what I pull out of this bag. Say what I say: mouse, children.**
14. Says the singular or irregular plural form of pictured nouns.	SLP: **Name the pictures in this puzzle as we put it together.** S: goose, mice, deer
Short-Term Goal: Uses both regular and irregular plural nouns	
15. Given a list of words, underlines the plural nouns.	SLP: **Look at this list of words. Now underline the ones that are plural.** S: Underlines *chicks*, *men*, and *children*.
16. Upon hearing the singular form of a noun, tells the regular or irregular plural form.	SLP: **What is the plural of *bus*? What is the plural of *tooth*?** S: **Buses, teeth**
17. Says singular and plural forms in complete sentences while describing pictures of surroundings.	SLP: **Use complete sentences to tell about these pictures.** S: **There are three ships on the ocean. The sheep are in the pasture.**
18. Chooses the appropriate plural or singular form in a written fill-in-the-blank activity.	SLP: **Write the correct singular or plural word to fill in the blank.** S: (writes) I picked up a *leaf*. A dentist cleans my *teeth*.

(continues)

Objectives	Examples
19. Judges whether spoken sentences are grammatical and corrects grammatically incorrect sentences.	SLP: **Decide if the sentences I say are grammatically correct, and change any incorrect sentences: There are three man at the table.** S: **Wrong. There are three men at the table.**
20. Uses singular and plural forms while retelling and creating stories.	SLP: **Retell a story that we just read using plurals correctly.**
21. Given a written paragraph, alters its meaning by changing singular nouns to plural nouns.	SLP: **Change the singular nouns to plural nouns in this article.** S: **A boy at the high school was a hero today. Two boys from the high school were heroes today.**
22. Writes the singular and plural forms in a paragraph about a given picture.	SLP: **Use correct singular and plural nouns as you write a paragraph to describe this painting.**
23. During a discussion about a given subject, uses the singular and plural forms of words.	SLP: **Tell me about the animals you saw today.** S: **We saw cows, fish, mice, and a horse.**

Copular (Linking) and Auxiliary (Helping) Verbs

Yearly Goal: *To develop correct use of copular (linking) and auxiliary (helping) verbs when listening, speaking, reading, and writing*

CCSS.ELA-LITERACY.L.K.1.B
CCSS.ELA-LITERACY.L.1.1.E
CCSS.ELA-LITERACY.L.3.1.D

Objectives	Examples
Short-Term Goal: Understands and imitates sentences using copular (linking) and auxiliary (helping) verbs	
1. Indicates when a sentence about an object sounds correct or incorrect.	SLP: **Listen. Does this sound right? Kyle my friend.** S: **No.**
2. Imitates sentences using present tense singular or plural auxiliary verbs to describe actions.	SLP: **Let's look around the classroom and see what's happening here. Say what I say: The children are listening. The bell is ringing.**
3. Imitates sentences using past tense singular or plural auxiliary verbs to describe actions.	SLP: **Say what I say about what was happening. The boy was swinging. The children were playing.**
4. Imitates sentences using present tense singular or plural copular verbs to describe objects or people.	SLP: **Let's describe some of the things in our classroom. Say what I say: The bear feels soft. The roses smell good. The globe is round.**
5. Imitates sentences using past tense singular or plural copular verbs to describe objects.	SLP: **Say what I say about these pictures of outdoor scenes. Susan looked at clouds. The clown sounded funny.**

Objectives	Examples
Short-Term Goal: Produces sentences using copular (linking) and auxiliary (helping) verbs	
6. Produces simple sentences using present tense singular or plural auxiliary verbs to describe action pictures.	SLP: **Tell about these pictures in your book and use *is* or *are*.** S: **The horse is running. They are sleeping.**
7. Produces sentences using present tense singular or plural copular verbs to describe pictures.	SLP: **Tell about animals you see on the mural. Use *looks* or *look*.** S: **The elephant looks huge. The jaguars look hungry.**
8. Produces sentences using past tense singular or plural auxiliary verbs to describe action pictures.	SLP: **We studied about floods. Tell about these photos of floods. Use the words *was* or *were*.** S: **The water was rising. The streets were flooding.**
9. Produces sentences using past tense singular or plural copular verbs to describe pictures.	SLP: **Tell about the pictures from the story *Stellaluna*. Use the words *was* or *were*.** S: **The owl was flying after the baby bats. Then all the baby bats were safe.**
Short-Term Goal: Chooses correct copular (linking) and auxiliary (helping) verbs or corrects errors during written assignments	
10. Chooses copular or auxiliary verbs to complete sentences.	SLP: **Choose *was* or *were* to complete the sentence: The boy _____ going home.** S: (writes) was
11. Corrects copular or auxiliary verbs used incorrectly in written sentences.	SLP: **Correct the helping and linking verb errors that you see on your work sheet.** S: (reads) They was writing an important part of our history. (writes) They were writing an important part of our history.
12. Corrects errors in auxiliary and copular verb usage when given an incorrectly written paragraph.	SLP: **Correct the helping or linking verbs written incorrectly in the paragraph written on the board: Potatoes is roots.** S: (writes) Potatoes are roots.
Short-Term Goal: Retells stories or relates life experiences using copular (linking) and auxiliary (helping) verbs	
13. Uses auxiliary and copular verbs to retell stories or events.	SLP: **We had a great nature walk. Tell about it, and use some linking and helping verbs.** S: **We were walking in the park. We saw a large tree. It looked very old.**
14. Uses future tense auxiliary and copular verbs to write sentences about pictures.	SLP: **We have seen a video about wild animals. Use helping verbs to write sentences about what the giraffes and bears will do next.** S: (writes) The giraffes will eat leaves from the trees. The bears will go into their caves.

(continues)

Objectives	Examples
15. Uses all forms of auxiliary and copular verbs to write a paragraph.	SLP: **Use helping and linking verbs in a paragraph about the circus that is in town.** S: **The circus has been coming to our town every year. The clowns were hiding in a little car. The lions and tigers were the best act.**
Short-Term Goal: Uses copular (linking) and auxiliary (helping) verbs in conversation and written assignments	
16. Uses copular and auxiliary verbs during conversation.	SLP: **Talk with others in your group about the story we read. Use the verbs that are written on the board: *was, were, seemed, felt, would, might.*** S: **The man felt tired. It seemed like the day should be finished. He might fall asleep early.**
17. Uses copular and auxiliary verbs when writing stories.	SLP: **Write a story about the science class field trip. How many linking and helping verbs did you use in your paragraph?**

Possessive Nouns

Yearly Goal: *To develop correct use of possessive nouns when listening, speaking, reading, and writing*

CCSS.ELA-LITERACY.RF.3.3.A
CCSS.ELA-LITERACY.L.K.4.B
CCSS.ELA-LITERACY.L.2.2.C

Objectives	Examples
1. Imitates the SLP's model as she labels possessions.	SLP: **We are going to pass these toys around in a circle. Say what I say. Caitlin's block. David's crayon.**
2. Locates objects described.	SLP: **Touch Natalie's shoe. Show me Charlie's desk.**
3. Points to the objects described in pictures.	SLP: **Look at these pictures and show me the police officer's hat. Touch the firefighter's truck.**
4. Answers questions about possessions using possessive nouns in single words.	SLP: **It's snack time! Whose cracker is this?** S: **Hayden's**
5. Labels objects as requested using possessive nouns in short phrases.	SLP: **Whose desk is this? Whose book is on the table?** S: **the teacher's desk, the librarian's book**
6. Completes a spoken sentence with a possessive noun given a sentence cue.	SLP: **Use a possessive noun to finish my sentence. The farmer has a tractor. The tractor is the _____.** S: **farmer's**

Objectives	Examples
7. Uses possessives in sentences to describe pictures.	SLP: **Use possessive nouns to describe what you see in this video.** S: **The bird's feathers are yellow. The fish's home is in the pond.**
8. Writes possessive nouns in short phrases to name objects and pictures requested.	SLP: **Write possessive nouns in short phrases to answer my questions. What is this?** S: (writes) the pioneer's covered wagon
9. Writes possessive nouns to fill in the blanks of sentences.	SLP: **Fill in the blanks with possessive nouns. The scientist does a lot of experiments. The _____ experiments are important.** S: (writes) scientist's
10. Corrects a written paragraph by changing inappropriately used possessive nouns.	SLP: **Correctly rewrite the sentence in this paragraph that has an incorrect possessive noun: The birds nest is finished.** S: (writes) The bird's nest is finished.
11. Writes a sentence using possessive nouns to describe surroundings.	SLP: **Write sentences using possessive nouns to describe the experiment we did today.** S: (writes) Jim's soap floated in the water. Nathan's rock sank.
12. Uses possessive nouns to retell a story.	SLP: **Retell the story we just read using possessive nouns.** S: **The story is about a girl's dream to become a ballet dancer. The girl's name is LaToya. LaToya's mother doesn't want her to take dancing lessons.**
13. Uses possessive nouns to relate personal life experiences.	SLP: **Use possessive nouns to tell about your family.** S: **My mother's name is Renee. I have two sisters. One's name is Bianca, and the other one's name is Jessica.**
14. Uses possessive nouns to write a story.	SLP: **Use possessive nouns in a written report to summarize the magazine article you read about the scientist's discovery.**

Comparatives and Superlatives

Yearly Goal: *To develop the understanding and correct use of comparatives and superlatives when listening, speaking, reading, and writing*

CCSS.ELA-LITERACY.L.3.1.G

Objectives	Examples
1. Answers comparison questions about two objects that differ along one dimension.	SLP: **Which triangle is bigger? Which square is smaller? Which rectangle is longer?** S: **The first triangle is bigger. The second square is smaller, and the first rectangle is longer.**
2. Answers comparison questions about three or more objects that differ along one dimension.	SLP: **Get into groups of three. Look at the people in your group. Who has the longest hair? Who is the tallest?** S: **I have the longest hair. Matt is the tallest.**
3. Answers *yes/no* questions comparing objects.	SLP: **Think about what we learned in our lesson. Is a lake bigger than an ocean?** S: **No.**
4. Tells whether spoken sentences comparing objects are grammatically correct and changes incorrect ones.	SLP: **Does this sound right? The airplane goes fastest than the helicopter.** S: **No. The airplane goes faster than the helicopter.**
5. Describes a picture by completing a sentence with a comparative or superlative.	SLP: **Finish this sentence using *bigger* or *biggest*. This redwood tree is the _____.** S: **biggest**
6. Makes picture comparisons by using comparatives and superlatives in sentences.	SLP: **Use comparatives or superlatives to compare these library books.** S: **My book is longer than this book. This is the tallest book on the shelf.**
7. Tells about family members, peers, and surroundings using comparatives and superlatives.	SLP: **Use comparatives and superlatives to compare the members in your group.** S: **Max is taller than Scott. Marsha has the longest hair.**
8. Chooses the appropriate comparatives or superlatives to complete written fill-in-the-blank tasks.	SLP: **On this work sheet, fill in the blank to complete these sentences with the correct comparative or superlative. New York has _____ people than Kansas.** S: (writes) more
9. Writes descriptive sentences about surroundings and objects using comparatives and superlatives.	SLP: **Use comparatives or superlatives when writing five sentences telling about the relay race.** S: **I ran faster than Marsha. Bart is the fastest runner in our class.**

Objectives	Examples
10. Uses comparatives and superlatives to write a paragraph about a given topic.	SLP: **Write a comparison paragraph using comparatives and superlatives telling how transportation in the 1800s was different from transportation today.**

Past Tense Verbs

Yearly Goal: *To develop understanding and correct use of past tense verbs when listening, speaking, reading, and writing*

CCSS.ELA-LITERACY.L.K.1.B
CCSS.ELA-LITERACY.L.1.1.E and L.3.1.E
CCSS.ELA-LITERACY.L.2.1.D and L.3.1.D

Note: Please refer to Appendix B ("Word Lists") for a list of the most common irregular past tense verbs.

Objectives	Examples
Short-Term Goal: Understands and uses regular past tense verbs	
1. Imitates actions and the regular past tense verbs that describe them.	SLP: **Let's play Follow the Leader. Do this. Clap your hands. Say "clapped."** S: (claps) **clapped**
2. After following directions, answers "What did you do?" using regular past tense verbs.	SLP: **It's fun to play Simon Says. Listen. Simon says, "Open the door." What did you do?** S: **Opened the door.**
3. After following directions, answers "What did you do?" using regular past tense verbs in sentences.	SLP: **Look at all these toys. You may choose one for a new game. Now listen. Hug the doll. What did you do? Say it in a sentence.** S: **I hugged the doll.**
4. States the regular past tense form of verbs requested.	SLP: **Let's have a "verb bee." Say the past tense of the verb I say: *walk*.** S: **Walked**
Short-Term Goal: Understands and uses irregular past tense verbs	
5. Imitates actions and the irregular past tense verbs that describe them.	SLP: **Everyone, let's make a circle. Stand up. Say what I say: stood up.** S: **Stood up**
6. After following directions, answers "What did you do?" using irregular past tense verbs.	SLP: **Listen carefully and follow the leader's directions. Cut the paper. What did you do?** S: **I cut the paper.**

(continues)

Objectives	Examples
7. Answers "What did you do?" questions with irregular past tense verbs in sentences after following directions.	SLP: **While we have a snack, we'll play a game. Use a sentence to answer my question. What did you eat? What did you drink?** S: **I ate the cookie. I drank my juice.**
8. States the irregular past tense form of verbs requested.	SLP: **Listen and fill in the blank. Today I throw; yesterday I _____.** S: **Threw**
Short-Term Goal: Uses both regular and irregular past tense verbs	
9. Discriminates correct and incorrect use of regular and irregular past tense verbs.	SLP: **Look at the driver. Which sentence is right? The man drived the car. The man drove the car.** S: **The man drove the car.**
10. Completes spoken sentences using regular and irregular past tense verbs to describe action pictures.	SLP: **Today we'll play a board game. Finish my sentence to describe this picture and take a turn at the game. Kim is riding a horse. She did the same thing yesterday. Yesterday she _____.** S: **Rode**
11. Answers "What did he/she/they do yesterday?" to describe action pictures using regular and irregular past tense verbs.	SLP: **Look at these pictures on the classroom calendar. What did they do on Monday?** S: **They drew a picture.**
12. Describes actions using regular and irregular past tense sentences.	SLP: **Use sentences to describe what a classmate did earlier today.** S: **Aaron scratched his nose. Mia read her book.**
13. Changes spoken sentences from present to past tense.	SLP: **Now that we've finished the story, change the sentence I say from the present to the past. The girl in our story is eating porridge.** S: **The girl in our story ate porridge.**
14. Uses regular and irregular past tense verbs to tell stories.	SLP: **Let's review our history lesson: What happened on March 6, 1836?** S: **The men inside the Alamo were defeated by the Mexican soldiers.**
15. Writes the regular or irregular past tense form of verbs requested.	SLP: **Get your paper and pencils. Write the past tense forms of the verbs I write on the board: *talk, sing, sit, jump, laugh.*** S: (writes) talked, sang, sat, jumped, laughed
16. Rewrites sentences in a paragraph by changing present tense verbs into their regular and irregular past tense forms.	SLP: **Rewrite these sentences from our lesson. Change sentences with present tense verbs to sentences with regular or irregular past tense verbs.** S: (reads) The girl sings a song every day. (writes) The girl sang a song every day.

Objectives	Examples
17. Uses regular and irregular past tense verbs to write sentences describing action pictures.	SLP: **Look at the pictures from our story. Write sentences using regular and irregular past tense verbs.** S: (writes) We spread peanut butter to make sandwiches, and Spot sat right between us. He begged for a bite.
18. Uses regular and irregular past tense verbs to talk about personal life experiences.	SLP: **Everyone has brought photos to show some things you did when you were younger. Use past tense verbs as you describe your picture.** S: **I held my father's hand when I crossed the street.**
19. Uses regular and irregular past tense verbs to write a story about a given event or personal life experience.	SLP: **Write about an experience you had during Spring Break. Then count the number of regular and irregular past tense verbs.**

Third Person Verbs

Yearly Goal: *To develop understanding and correct use of third person verbs when listening, speaking, reading, and writing*

CCSS.ELA-LITERACY.L.K.4.B
CCSS.ELA-LITERACY.L.1.1.C

Objectives	Examples
1. Imitates sentences describing object actions using third person verbs.	SLP: **When it's your turn, say what I say. A car goes. A pencil writes. A drawer opens.**
2. Indicates whether third person verbs are used correctly or incorrectly in spoken sentences.	SLP: **Let's play a listening game. Everyone gets a turn. Does this sound right? A bird fly high.** S: **No.**
3. Uses third person verbs to fill in the end of spoken sentences.	SLP: **Did you like the story? Finish my sentence about the story. The Gingerbread Boy is running. All through the book he ______.** S: **Runs**
4. Acts out and guesses actions using sentences containing third person verbs.	SLP: **Today we'll act out what several animals can do. Listen.** (Crows like a rooster.) **Tell me what a rooster does.** S: **A rooster crows.**
5. Uses third person verbs to answer "What does he/she/it do?" about pictures.	SLP: **Here are pictures of women and men working. This is a firefighter. What does a firefighter do? Use a sentence.** S: **A firefighter puts out fires.**

(continues)

Objectives	Examples
6. Uses third person verbs to tell about family members and friends.	SLP: **You brought some photos of your family. Tell about what your family members like to do.** S: **My dad likes to go fishing. My sister loves mystery stories.**
7. Writes third person verbs to fill in sentence blanks.	SLP: **Finish my sentences by writing third person verbs. This woman is running fast. Every day she _____.** S: (writes) runs
8. Rewrites a paragraph by correcting inappropriately used third person verbs.	SLP: **Read this paragraph and circle all the incorrect verbs. Then rewrite the paragraph correctly.**
9. Uses third person verbs in sentences to tell about events taking place.	SLP: **Let's watch the soccer match. Use correct third person verbs to tell what each player does.** S: **Don kicks the soccer ball down the field.**
10. Uses third person verbs to write a story about a sequence of events.	SLP: **Write about what happens when you go to the dentist. Then reread your paragraph and count the third person verbs.** S: (writes) The dental hygienist puts a bib around my neck. Then she cleans my teeth. **There are two third person verbs in my paragraph.**

Infinitives

Yearly Goal: *To develop understanding and correct use of the infinitive* to + verb *when listening, speaking, reading, and writing*

Objectives	Examples
1. Tells if a sentence that uses or should use the infinitive *to + verb* is correct or incorrect.	SLP: **Look carefully at this picture and listen. Does this sound right or wrong? Emily wants run.** S: **Wrong.**
2. Uses an infinitive *to + verb* in a phrase to answer questions about objects.	SLP: **Look around the room to see objects that we use in our classroom work. Here's an eraser. Why do we need erasers?** S: **We need erasers to erase the board.**
3. Uses the infinitive *to + verb* to complete a sentence about a picture.	SLP: **Look at these pictures of children having a good time. Finish my sentence with an infinitive. Benjamin likes _____.** S: **To run**
4. Uses the infinitive *to + verb* when shown a picture and asked what the person likes or needs to do.	SLP: **Look at the picture of Jack having a good time. What does Jack like to do?** S: **Jack likes to climb trees.**

Objectives	Examples
5. Uses the infinitive *to* + *verb* when asked about job responsibilities.	SLP: **Look at our classroom duty chart. Tell what Abdul needs to do every day.** S: **Abdul needs to erase the chalkboard.**
6. Uses the infinitive *to* + *verb* to tell the function or purpose of objects.	SLP: **Let's think about purposes for parts of animals' bodies. Tell the purpose of a fish's gills.** S: **Fish need gills to breathe.**
7. Writes sentences containing the infinitive *to* + *verb* when telling about likes, dislikes, or things that must be done.	SLP: **Write your answer to this question: Would you like to do what Columbus did?** S: (writes) Yes, I'd like to sail around the world.
8. Uses the infinitive *to* + *verb* when writing a paragraph or story.	SLP: **Here is your topic. Write a paragraph that tells what we need to do to have world peace.**

Future Tense Verbs

Yearly Goal: *To develop understanding and correct use of future tense verbs when listening, speaking, reading, and writing.*

CCSS.ELA-LITERACY.L.K.1.B
CCSS.ELA-LITERACY.L.1.1.E and L.3.1.E

Objectives	Examples
1. Indicates when a sentence about a future activity is stated correctly or incorrectly.	SLP: **Listen carefully to what I say. Does this sentence sound right? The police officer will direct traffic last night.** S: **No.**
2. Points to action pictures that correspond with spoken future tense sentences.	SLP: **Look at all the giraffes in this mural. With this pointer, touch the tip to "The giraffe will reach up into the tree to eat the leaves."**
3. Imitates future tense sentences about pictures or actions about to happen.	SLP: **Let's talk about plans for the day. Say what I say: You will make kites today after school.**
4. Produces future tense sentences to describe action pictures in answer to "What will happen?"	SLP: **Look at this picture. What do you think will happen if the girl puts the seeds in the ground?** S: **The flowers will grow.**
5. Tells about activities about to happen using future tense sentences.	SLP: **Tell your partner about plans for this school day.** S: **First, we will have a spelling test. Then we will all go outside for Field Day.**
6. Retells a story about what will happen next to the characters using future tense verbs.	SLP: **Did you like the Goldilocks fairy tale? Tell what you think will happen next.** S: **Goldilocks will tell her mother all about the bears' house. The bears will eat their porridge and will remember to lock the door the next time they leave.**

(continues)

Objectives	Examples
7. Writes future tense verbs in a fill-in-the-blank activity.	SLP: **The video was about volcanoes. Use future tense verbs to fill in sentence blanks. The lava from a volcano is so hot it can burn anything in its path. It _____ trees and homes.** S: (writes) will burn
8. Writes predictions about what will happen next using future tense verbs.	SLP: **Do you like the story we're reading about George Washington? What do you think he will do next? Write your answer.** S: (writes) He will lead his troops across the river.
9. Writes an ending to a story using future tense verbs.	SLP: **On the video, we saw bears looking for food in the fall. Write what will happen next.** S: (writes) The bears will look for a place to hibernate. They will choose a safe place.
10. Writes a story using future tense verbs.	SLP: **Write a story about what you think will happen if we all begin taking better care of our environment.**

Articles

Yearly Goal: *To develop understanding and correct use of the articles* a, an, *and* the *when listening, speaking, reading, and writing*

CCSS.ELA-LITERACY.RF.K.3.C
CCSS.ELA-LITERACY.L.1.1.H

Objectives	Examples
1. When looking at a variety of objects, points to the correct one when described by the SLP with an article and a noun.	SLP: **Point to the one I am talking about: a bear, an elephant, the giraffe.**
2. When shown various objects, imitates the SLP's model using the articles *a*, *an*, and *the*.	SLP: **Look at what I pull out of the box and say what I say: a truck, an apple, the desk.**
3. Correctly reads the sight words *a*, *an*, and *the*.	SLP: **Read these words aloud as I show you the cards.** S: **A, an, the**
4. Uses the articles *a* and *the* appropriately when shown pictures and asked to talk about them.	SLP: **Use the articles *a* and *the* to answer questions about these pictures. What did Jen get for her birthday?** S: **A bike**
5. Uses the articles *a* and *the* in structured sentences to tell about pictures.	SLP: **Tell me what you see. Begin with *I see*.** S: **I see a bus. I see the train.**

Objectives	Examples
6. Given various phrases and sentences, judges the grammatical correctness of the use of articles.	SLP: **Listen to my sentence. If it sounds right, put a mark by the happy face. If it sounds wrong, put a mark by the sad face. I see a hammer. He is using drill.** S: Puts a mark by the happy face and then by the sad face.
7. When verbally given a list of nouns, chooses the appropriate article *a* or *an* to precede each noun.	SLP: **Here are two cards. One says *a* and one says *an*. Listen to the words I say. Hold up the card that comes before my word: *apple*.** S: (holds up) an
8. When describing a picture containing a variety of items, includes articles in complete sentences.	SLP: **Who do you see on our community helper poster?** S: **I see a police officer, a firefighter, and an ambulance driver.**
9. Includes articles in structured conversation.	SLP: **Draw a picture about our sink-or-float experiment and tell me about it.** S: **I put a rock and an apple in the water. The rock sank.**
10. Uses the articles *a*, *an*, and *the* correctly in conversation.	SLP: **Use *a*, *an*, and *the* correctly while we talk about this chapter.** S: **The boy wants to be a baseball player.**
11. In a written activity, completes sentences with an appropriate noun to correspond with the preceding article.	SLP: **Fill in the blanks on this work sheet with nouns that go with the articles: Jerry went to the zoo and saw an _____.** S: (writes) ostrich
12. Uses the articles *a*, *an*, and *the* correctly in written stories and reports.	SLP: **Use articles correctly when writing your report.**

Conjunctions and Transition Words

Yearly Goal: *To establish understanding and use of conjunctions and transition words when listening, speaking, reading, and writing*

CCSS.ELA-LITERACY.W.6.2.C
CCSS.ELA-LITERACY.L.1.1.G
CCSS.ELA-LITERACY.L.1.6
CCSS.ELA-LITERACY.L.5.1.E

Note: Please refer to Appendix B ("Word Lists") for a list of conjunctions and transition words.

Objectives	Examples
Short-Term Goal: Uses frequently occurring conjunctions to indicate simple relationships	
1. Points to two objects or pictures when the SLP gives a direction with the conjunction *and*.	SLP: **Touch the apple and the banana.**
2. Uses the conjunction *and* in phrases or sentences to name two objects.	SLP: **What two toys do you want?** S: **Baby and blanket. I want the blocks and the puzzle.**
3. Tells about pictured actions of two people using the conjunction *but*.	SLP: **Tell me about Sara and Jan. Use the word *but* in your sentence.** S: **Sara is swinging, but Jan is running.**
4. Finishes phrases containing associated items.	SLP: **Finish my sentence and use *and*. (1) Two animals that live on a farm are a cow _____.** **Finish my question and use *or*. (2) Do you like to go to the beach _____?** S: **(1) and a pig, (2) or the mountains**
5. Makes two sentences from a spoken sentence containing the conjunctions *or, and, but*.	SLP: **Listen. Lakes are big, but oceans are bigger. Make that into two sentences.** S: **Lakes are big. Oceans are bigger.**
6. Makes two spoken sentences into one sentence by adding the conjunction *because, or, and, but*.	SLP: **Choose from *because, or, and, but* to make my two sentences into one. She made a good grade on her test. She studied hard.** S: **She made a good grade on her test because she studied hard.**
7. Describes a picture using sentences joined by a conjunction, such as *because, but, or, and, so*.	SLP: **Use *because, but, or, and, so* to tell about two things that you see in this picture.** S: **The horse is thirsty, so he is drinking from the creek.**

Objectives	Examples
8. Chooses the correct conjunction to finish a spoken fill-in-the-blank activity, such as *and, but, or, because, so, if, while, until.*	SLP: **Choose from the list of conjunctions written on the board to fill in the blank in my sentence. He likes vanilla ice cream, _____ I prefer chocolate. Would you like chips _____ french fries with your hamburger?** S: **But, or**
9. Finishes a sentence correctly with the correlative conjunctions *either/or, neither/nor.*	SLP: **Let's make some plans for the Field Day. Finish my sentences. For activities, we can have either a jump rope contest _____. Neither Patrick _____ wants to do the relay race.** S: **Or a softball throw; nor Justin**
10. Creates a sentence using a given conjunction.	SLP: **Throw a beanbag at one of the cards taped to the wall. Read the conjunction and use it in a sentence about birds.** S: Hits the conjunction words *because* and *so*. **Birds can fly because they have wings. Birds build a nest so they can lay their eggs.**
11. Relates personal experiences using conjunctions.	SLP: **Use at least two of the conjunctions listed on the board as you tell us about your summer.** S: **We went to the beach because it's our favorite place. We could not go out in the sun until we put sunscreen on.**
12. Makes two written sentences from one longer sentence.	SLP: **Read each long sentence. Now use it to write two short sentences. The plant died because we didn't water it.** S: (writes) The plant died. We didn't water it.
13. Uses a conjunction to combine two sentences into one written sentence.	SLP: **Listen to my two sentences about our science lesson, and then write them as one sentence using a conjunction. Hydrogen is in the air. Oxygen is in the air.** S: (writes) Hydrogen and oxygen are in the air.
Short-Term Goal: Uses transition words to clarify relationships among ideas	
14. Shows cause–effect relations in spoken or written sentences using transition words, such as *because of, as a result, due to, if–then, in order to, since, consequently, therefore.*	SLP: **Our class enjoyed the air show. Write a short paragraph about the day. Use the transition phrase *as a result*.** S: (writes) I love airplanes. As a result, I went to the air show to learn more about the history of airplanes.
15. Writes cohesive narratives and descriptions that are ordered logically or temporally and that are connected with time relations using transition words, such as *after that, after awhile, as soon as, finally, meanwhile, until, when, soon, shortly.*	SLP: **Learning to do new things is fun. Write about a time when you mastered a skill. Use the transition phrase *after that*.** S: (writes) I was afraid of water until I took sailing lessons. After that, I always felt safe in sailboats because I was a seasoned sailor!

(continues)

Objectives	Examples
16. Writes cohesive narratives and descriptions that are ordered logically or temporally and that are connected with descriptive relations using transition words, such as *besides, for example, for instance, in addition to.*	SLP: **We're learning to make transitions in our writing. In your paragraph use the transition phrase *for example*.** S: (writes) I have choices about what to do this weekend. For example, I could have friends over, go to a movie, or go to the park.
17. Writes cohesive narratives and descriptions that are ordered logically or temporally and that are connected with *then relations* using transition words, such as *then, next, such as, finally, eventually, also, as soon as, first, second, third.*	SLP: **I wrote some transition words on the board to help you show changes or shifts in your ideas. Write about the steps in frying an egg.** S: (writes) First, get out a skillet and an egg. Then pour a little oil in the skillet and turn on the burner. Crack the egg into a skillet and cook. Finally, flip it over and cook briefly. When done, transfer the egg to a plate. Enjoy!
18. Writes cohesive narratives and descriptions that are ordered logically or temporally and that are connected with *comparative relations* using transition words to indicate comparisons, such as *however, in comparison, in contrast, likewise, nevertheless, on the other hand, similarly, yet.*	SLP: **Write about a time when you had a surprise. Use transition words.** S: (writes) We Scouts were surprised at how strenuous it was to climb to the top of the hill. Nevertheless, we had a great time. We plan to do it again!
19. Writes cohesive narratives and descriptions that are ordered logically or temporally and that are connected with *transition words* that indicate summaries or concluding sentences using transition words, such as *in conclusion, as I have said, therefore, to summarize.*	SLP: **Today when you are writing, pay special attention to your transition to your conclusion. Write a sentence to summarize and conclude your thoughts about whales.** S: (writes) In conclusion, whales are not only the largest animals in the sea but also highly intelligent. Whales are amazing creatures!

Modal Auxiliaries

Yearly Goal: *To develop understanding and correct use of modal auxiliaries when speaking, reading, and writing*

CCSS.ELA-LITERACY.L.4.1.C

Note. Refer to Appendix B ("Word Lists") for a list of modal auxiliaries.

Objectives	Examples
1. Uses the modal auxiliary *can* in sentences to tell about people, animals, and objects.	SLP: **Let's play a team game. Use the word *can* to answer this question. Steve can jump rope. What can he do?** S: **He can jump rope.**

Objectives	Examples
2. Uses the modal auxiliary *may* to ask permission.	SLP: **When we ask permission, we use the word *may*. Ask to use the pencil sharpener.** S: **May I sharpen my pencil?**
3. Uses the modal auxiliary *will* to predict outcomes of short stories or to tell about the future.	SLP: **Look at the calendar and tell something our class *will* do on Friday.** S: **We will go on a field trip.**
4. Uses the modal *must* to discuss realistic situations and the way events have to be done.	SLP: **Your show-and-tell airplane is beautiful. Explain the steps to follow to make it. Use *must*.** S: **You must let the paint dry before you add the propellers.**
5. Uses the modal auxiliary *would* to discuss what the student would do in various situations.	SLP: **Use the word *would* to tell what you would do if you forgot to bring your lunch to school.** S: **I would ask my teacher if I could call my mom to bring it.**
6. Uses the modal auxiliaries *could* or *might* in sentences to discuss future events or give possible solutions to problems.	SLP: **Use the modal auxiliaries *could* or *might* to answer this question: What could you be when you grow up?** S: **I could be a teacher. I might be a firefighter.**
7. Uses the modal auxiliary *should* to talk about social situations.	SLP: **Look at these picture scenes. Use *should* to answer this question: What should you do if there is a fire drill?** S: **You should line up quickly and quietly.**
8. Retells stories or relates personal experiences using modal auxiliaries: *can, could, may, might, shall, should, will, would, must.*	SLP: **When you give your report, use modal auxiliaries when telling us what each athlete in the Olympics must do to win.** S: **An athlete must practice hard and keep fit.**
9. Fills in the blank by writing the correct modal auxiliaries: *can, could, may, might, shall, should, will, would, must.*	SLP: **Look at the modal auxiliaries on the board. Choose from the list to fill in the blank. The students _____ study the spelling words before the test.** S: (writes) should
10. Writes modal auxiliaries correctly in sentences to answer questions or solve problems.	SLP: **We had a noisy thunderstorm this morning. What *might* cause a thunderstorm? Use modal auxiliaries when you write your answer.** S: (writes) When warm and cold air come together, it might cause a thunderstorm.
11. Writes all modal auxiliaries correctly in paragraphs, reports, or stories, giving explanations or solutions to problems.	SLP: **The man in this newspaper article was convicted of robbing three banks. Write about what might or could happen next. Use *might, could, may* in your paragraph.** S: (writes) The robber could be arrested. He might go to court. The judge may decide to put him in jail.

(continues)

Objectives	Examples
12. Uses the context of a situation to answer indirect questions that contain the modal auxiliary *can't*.	SLP: **Look at this picture. Mom has her arms full of groceries. She says, "Can't you open the door?" What does she mean?** S: **Open the door.**
13. Uses the context of a situation to answer indirect questions that contain the modal auxiliary *will*.	SLP: **Look at this picture of a family room. The room is littered with toys. Father says, "Will you pick it up now?" What does he mean?** S: **Pick up the toys.**
14. Uses the context of a situation to answer indirect questions that contain the modal auxiliary *must*.	SLP: **Suppose your mother is talking on the phone and you turn on loud music. She says to you, "Must you play that music now?" What does she mean?** S: **Turn off the music.**
15. Uses the context of a situation to answer indirect questions that contain the modal auxiliary *should*.	SLP: **It's important to know what's happening around us in order to understand messages. Suppose it's very cold outside, and your brother says, "Should you wear a coat?" What does he mean?** S: **Wear a coat.**

Complex Sentences

Yearly Goal: *To establish the understanding and correct use of complex sentences when listening, speaking, reading, and writing*

CCSS.ELA-LITERACY.L.3.1.H
CCSS.ELA-LITERACY.L.3.1.I

Note: Understanding and using complex sentences are dependent on children's cognitive awareness of a variety of conceptual relationships (Owens, 1999). These are expressed with different types of conjunctions and transition words. See the list of conjunctions and transition words in Appendix B.

Objectives	Examples
1. Follows directions stated in complex sentences containing conjunctions, such as *what*, *when*, *so*, *because*, *but*, and *if*.	SLP: **Today we get to play a fun listening game with paper and pencil. Don't start until I say *go*. If you are a boy, draw a circle on your page. Go.**
2. Chooses the pictures described by complex sentences.	SLP: **These picture pairs are almost the same. Listen. Circle this picture: The man played football although he didn't have a uniform.** S: Circles the picture of a man without a uniform playing football.
3. Indicates whether or not complex sentences describing pictures are grammatical.	SLP: **Pretend you are a complex sentence detective. Does this sound right or wrong? Because he got the most votes, he won the election.** S: **Right**

Objectives	Examples
4. Uses complex sentences while participating in a role-play activity.	SLP: **It's fun to role-play. Pretend you're taking a long road trip across the desert. Describe what you are doing and what you see. Use complex sentences.** S: **Since we've been driving for a long time, I'm getting bored. I'll look for tall cactus. Wow! I see a cactus that's taller than a bus.**
5. Uses a conjunction to complete a fill-in-the-blank complex sentence describing a picture.	SLP: **Look carefully at these pictures to find causes and their effects. Fill in the blank. _____ Alice was ill, she went home.** S: **Because**
6. Writes two base sentences from one longer complex sentence.	SLP: **Can you discover two sentences in this long sentence? The man who is directing traffic is a police officer. Write them on your paper.** S: (writes) The man is directing traffic. The man is a police officer.
7. Writes one complex sentence by combining two shorter sentences.	SLP: **Rewrite these two sentences into one sentence: The building burned. The building was the library.** S: (writes) The building that burned was the library.
8. Uses complex sentences in a written paragraph to add variety to sentence structure.	SLP: **Today we will work on increasing variety in the types of sentences we use. In your paragraph use at least two complex sentences. Tell how you feel about the changes in the school library.**

Passive Sentences

Yearly Goal: *To develop the understanding and correct use of passive sentences when listening, speaking, reading, and writing*

CCSS.ELA-LITERACY.L.8.1.B

Objectives	Examples
1. Answers true or false questions about actions described with passive sentences.	SLP: **Let's watch one another's actions during PE. Listen and answer true or false. The soccer ball was kicked by Ethan.**
2. Chooses the picture described by a passive sentence.	SLP: **Which picture matches this sentence? The book was given to Carrie by her big sister.** S: Points to a picture of the big sister giving Carrie a book.
3. Answers questions about the actor and agent in passive sentences.	SLP: **In the story, Paul was pushed by Tim. Who did the pushing?** S: **Tim**

(continues)

Objectives	Examples
4. Tells if the meanings of sentence pairs are the same or different.	SLP: **Do these two sentences have the same meaning or a different meaning? Birds are protected by feathers. Birds protect feathers.** S: **Different**
5. Rearranges scrambled groupings of phrases into passive sentences that make sense.	SLP: **Here is a scrambled sentence. Arrange these phrases into a sentence: was chewed by the dog the bone.** S: **The bone was chewed by the dog.**
6. Orally changes passive sentences into active sentences with the same meaning.	SLP: **Change this passive sentence about forests into an active sentence that means the same thing: The tree was cut down by the lumberjack.** S: **The lumberjack cut down the tree.**
7. Orally describes action pictures using passive sentences.	SLP: **Use at least one passive sentence when you describe how the Industrial Revolution changed the United States.** S: **Our country was changed from an agricultural nation to an industrial nation by the Industrial Revolution.**
8. After reading a passive sentence, identifies the actor and agent.	SLP: **Read aloud each passive sentence. Identify the actor and agent in the sentence.** S: **The car was driven by Dad. Dad was the actor. The car was the agent.**
9. Writes the active sentence that means the same as a given passive sentence.	SLP: **Our play review arrived! As you read it, find the passive sentences and write them as active sentences.** S: (reads) The lead part was played by Monica. (writes) Monica played the lead part.
10. Understands that active sentences are generally clearer, but passive sentences can show what is more important than the doer of the action.	SLP: **At times passive sentences are stronger. They can make meanings clearer. Change this active sentence to passive: They grow wheat in many states.** S: **Wheat is grown in many states.**
11. Edits own paragraphs to use active sentences as much as possible to add directness and forcefulness.	SLP: **Edit your story's first draft. Change most of your passive sentences to active sentences. Start with your first sentence: I am called JJ by my family.** S: (writes) My family calls me JJ.
12. Uses at least one passive sentence in a written story or paragraph about a personal experience or event.	SLP: **Write a story about yesterday's trip to the museum. Include at least one passive sentence.** S: (writes) Our trip was delayed by a thunderstorm.

Unit 4

Critical Thinking for Language and Communication

- **Gathering Information**
- **Recalling Information From Short- and Long-Term Memory**
- **Making Sense of Information Gathered**
- **Applying and Evaluating Information in New Situations**
- **Thinking About Your Own Thinking**

The importance that education places on critical and creative thought affects how speech–language pathologists (SLPs) plan and implement intervention. *Thinking* is defined as the operating skill that uses intelligence for a purpose (de Bono, 1994). Some of the purposes are recalling, reasoning, judging, analyzing, inferring, imagining, and problem solving.

Critical thinking is basic to language and communication and all learning. According to Owens (2010, p. 354), "Critical thinking is the collection, manipulation and application of information to problem solving. Language is an integral part of this process." Therefore, children with language impairments may find it difficult to organize information, make decisions, and make metalinguistic judgments.

Buttrill, Niizawa, Biemer, Takahashi, and Hearn (1989) divided critical thinking training into three groups of general thinking, problem solving, and high-level thinking. Observation, description, development of concepts, comparisons and contrasts, hypothesis, and generalization are all part of general thinking. Problem solving includes analyzing, developing options, predicting outcomes, and critiquing the decision. Doing deductive and inductive reasoning, solving analogies, and understanding relationships are included in high-level thinking. This hierarchy of thinking skills is similar to that put forth by Benjamin Bloom in *Taxonomy of Educational Objectives* (Bloom, 1956). In both, the tasks become increasingly more abstract and require greater reliance on linguistic input.

Because higher level thinking skills are grounded in language, students with language impairments often require specific instruction in critical thinking, from the most basic tasks of naming, matching, and comparing to the more abstract skills of analyzing, predicting, and evaluating. Nelson (2010, p. 410) noted that children form concepts about their own intelligence, strengths, and abilities. Children who see their thinking and learning abilities as static are less likely to put energy into learning than will children who think of their intellectual abilities as open to change. Researchers have suspected that the breakdowns begin in the areas of processing and metacognition.

Description of Contents

The objectives in this unit are organized according to the Model of Thinking by Costa and Lowery (1989, p. 23). This model serves as a basis for the development of activities and questions that will help the student perform the intellectual functions represented in the model. This unit includes the following sections.

Gathering Information. There is an intake of data through the senses. Input goals target activating the senses to gather information in open and flexible ways. Gathering information involves using the senses: observing, listening, feeling, touching, tasting, and smelling.

Recalling Information From Short- and Long-Term Memory. We retrieve information from short- and long-term memory storage. Retrieval objectives target drawing from the student the concepts, information, feelings, or experiences acquired in the past and stored in long- or short-term memory. Retrieval involves defining, naming, identifying, pointing to, matching, completing, and so on.

Making Sense of Information Gathered. We make sense (meaning) of the information, processing it into meaningful relationships by comparing it with or relating it to information stored in short- and long-term memory. Processing involves organizing, categorizing, comparing, contrasting, and analyzing.

Applying and Evaluating Information in New Situations. We then apply the meaningful relationships to new or novel situations. It is in this area that the most complex thinking activities take place. Processing objectives target thinking creatively and hypothetically by using imagination, applying a value system, or making a critical judgment or evaluation. Output involves predicting, inferring, and generalizing.

Thinking About Your Own Thinking. Thinking about our own thinking is known as *metacognition*. Objectives for metacognition target knowing what one knows and what needs to be known to achieve a goal, assessing the success or failure of problem-solving strategies, and allowing patterns to emerge. Metacognition involves observing and describing one's own thinking and the thinking observed in others, expressing joy in thinking, and seeing oneself as a thinker.

Gathering Information

Yearly Goal: *To gather information through the senses: observing, listening, touching, tasting, and smelling*

Objectives	Examples
Short-Term Goal: Perceives a situation or information in open, flexible ways	
1. Develops an awareness of using the senses to gather information through sight, hearing, touch, taste, and smell.	SLP: **We have five senses that help us gather information about the world. Let's see what our senses can help us learn about this apple by what we see, smell, touch, taste, and hear.** S: **I see that it is red and roundish. It has a stem. Its skin feels smooth. It smells fruity. It tastes sweet, and it sounds crunchy when I take a bite.**
2. Observes a situation or collects information in a systematic way without judging it.	SLP: **What information did you gather from your experiment and what you observed?** S: **We planted a few seeds in two small flowerpots with soil. We watered pot 1 and placed it in a sunny spot. We did not water pot 2 and placed it in a dark cupboard. After a week we compared the pots. Pot 1 had a tiny plant with two leaves. Pot 2 had no plant and dry soil. We found out that flower seeds must have water and sunlight to grow.**
3. After gathering information, considers personal preferences and feelings when choosing alternatives.	SLP: **You want to grow flowers. Do you have a personal goal in mind about gardening?** S: **My personal goal is to learn to grow flowers in our front yard this spring. Flowers must have sun and water. Our front yard is very sunny, and there's a water hose connection there. I think I'll be able to grow flowers at home!**
4. Gathers resources before getting started on a project.	SLP: **Ask yourself, "What materials will I need to grow flowers, and how will I get them?"** S: **I will need seeds, a spade to dig the soil, flower fertilizer, and a water sprinkler. I can borrow the tools from my grandfather.**
5. Increases understanding of others' contributions by listening actively and openly.	SLP: **Your team has a large sheet of paper to draw your mural. Be sure to discuss and use ideas from each team member.** S: Each student contributes ideas, listens actively and openly to the ideas of others, makes a plan, and works with the team to create the mural.

Recalling Information From Short- and Long-Term Memory

Yearly Goal: *To recall and recognize given information and ideas in the approximate form in which they were learned*

CCSS.ELA-LITERACY.W.1.8–W.5.8

Objectives	Examples
1. Points to, recalls, matches, or tells about specific details or events.	SLP: **We finished the story. Now look at the picture on page 14. What do you see in the picture to help you recall the Princess's feelings?** S: **The Princess has received a valuable gift of 10 fine horses from an unknown giver. She feels puzzled and amazed. "Why did I receive these beautiful horses?" she wonders.**
2. Identifies, names, counts, or lists feelings, experiences, or information acquired in the past.	SLP: **Study this page that shows many facial expressions. So far today, which of these feelings have you had? List them and give the reasons you felt as you did.** S: (writes) Angry when my dog snatched my lunch bag. Sad when I heard the news report. Relieved when I made a good grade. Happy when my friend and I shared lunch.
3. Answers *wh-* questions about given information (e.g., who, what, where, when, which, how, or why).	SLP: **Columbus died in Spain in 1506 without ever realizing the great scope of what he achieved. What was it that he achieved?** S: **He discovered the New World for Europe. The riches that came from his discovery helped make Spain the wealthiest and most powerful nation on Earth.**
4. Describes or defines concepts and information acquired in the past.	SLP: **What did we learn last year on our visit to Turtle Island that helped us enjoy our return to the island today?** S: **Last year we learned that the turtles on Turtle Island came to the island because the food supplies in their old habitat were shrinking. They found refuge on Turtle Island. We felt excited today when we saw healthy turtles!**

Making Sense of Information Gathered

Yearly Goal: *To make sense out of ideas and concepts by breaking them apart to show relationships through categorizing, comparing and contrasting, sequencing, summarizing, analyzing, and interpreting*

CCSS.ELA-LITERACY.SL.K.5–CCSS.ELA-LITERACY.SL.7.5
CCSS.ELA-LITERACY.SL.5.2–CCSS.ELA-LITERACY.SL.7.2
CCSS.ELA-LITERACY.RH.6-8.8

Note: Refer to Appendix C for visual organizers.

Objectives	Examples
1. Organizes objects or pictures into categories.	SLP: **See how many ways you can organize these pictures of animals into different categories.** S: **I organized them into mammals and reptiles, wild and tame, small and large.**
2. Relates new information to known information.	SLP: **Here is a new puzzle for your group to work. What did you learn the last time you worked a puzzle that you can use again?** S: **I learned to look for all the corner pieces first, then the pieces with straight edges.**
3. Illustrates a story, story setting, or character by drawing pictures.	SLP: **We've seen the movie. Now draw a picture about the conflict between Thomas and Ben.** S: Draws picture of two boys who both want the same toy.
4. Compares two people or objects by telling how they're alike or different.	SLP: **After you read the story, explain to your partner ways that Noah and John are alike.** S: **Noah and John are alike because they both have huge appetites. They're the same age and both have younger sisters. Both love to run.**
5. Classifies objects, events, or ideas.	SLP: **Organize these magazines on the four shelves. Then explain how you chose the groups.** S: Groups magazines on shelves by soccer, football, baseball, and tennis.
6. Arranges information from a classroom activity into a logical sequence.	SLP: **Arrange in order these pictures of the steps you followed to put together your gingerbread house.**
7. Summarizes or paraphrases basic information. (See Appendix C for visual organizers.)	SLP: **You know how to use visual organizers and webs to summarize information. Make an organizer to summarize stages in your life.** S: **A sequential web would begin at my birth and end with this year. Each circle on my web would show a major event of that period.**

(continues)

Objectives	Examples
8. Organizes parts of a story or experience into logical sequences.	SLP: **Experiment and have fun with your thinking. How many ways can you organize the story?** S: **I could list the themes, the sequence of main events, the main character's feelings, or the contrasts in the story.**
9. Compares and contrasts words, characters, places, topics, and themes to identify similarities and differences.	SLP: **Compare and contrast the Troll and Big Billy Goat from *The Three Billy Goats Gruff.*** S: **Both were big and strong with strong voices, but Big Billy Goat had sharp horns. He used them to throw Troll into the river.**
10. Shows understanding of the main idea and the supporting details of material heard, seen, or read.	SLP: **Explain to your partner the main idea of this story. She will give supporting details.** S1: **The story was mostly about Adam, who had to grow up quickly.** S2: **Adam's big challenge came when he had to help defend his town against the British redcoats. At first he was terrified, but he discovered that he had the courage he needed.**
11. Distinguishes between fact and opinion.	SLP: **Debate with your discussion group whether each statement on the board is fact or opinion.** S: **Facts: Smoking is bad for your health. My dad is taller than your dad. Opinions: My mom is the best mom in the world. Dogs make better pets than turtles.**
12. Takes apart and analyzes the meanings and intents of words, expressions, and graphics.	SLP: **How many ways can you define a word?** S: **Tell about its name, category, use, attributes, and associated people or places.**
13. Describes cause-and-effect relationships.	SLP: **Discuss the effect that being born into a skating family had on Emma Johnston, the famous speed skater.** S: **Emma's family encouraged her from the time she first skated at age 3. Their cheers encouraged her to practice hard and be her best. She was competitive like her siblings, and she loved skating.**
14. Interprets the author's purpose (e.g., to entertain, describe, inform, persuade) and style (e.g., short sentences, much use of similes and metaphors).	SLP: **You read the book *"Stand Back," Said the Elephant, "I'm Going to Sneeze!"* to the kindergartners. Why do you think the author wrote the story? Talk about how you know.** S: **We decided that the author's purpose was to make us laugh. The kindergartners laughed out loud! They wanted to see every picture. That made them laugh even more.**

Applying and Evaluating Information in New Situations

Yearly Goal: *To bring together parts of information to form a new whole by predicting, inferring, and generalizing*

CCSS.ELA-LITERACY.CCRA.SL.2–CCSS.ELA-LITERACY.SL.3.2
CCSS.ELA-LITERACY.SL.1.2–CCSS.ELA-LITERACY.SL.5.2

Note: See Appendix C for visual organizers.

Objectives	Examples
1. Makes predictions about what will happen next in a story or situation.	SLP: **Take turns telling a story using these three sequence pictures. The fourth picture is missing. What could it be about?** S: **Hannah's friend Sarah will return from Italy. She will have a party to welcome her home. Hannah will send out invitations to the party. The fourth picture could be everyone having fun at the party.**
2. Draws inferences from implied information in situations, texts, electronic media, or advertisements.	SLP: **Suppose you are in a noisy cafeteria. Suddenly it gets quiet. What do you think could have happened? Brainstorm possibilities.** S: **Some of our ideas: (1) The principal and two firemen went onto the stage. (2) It thundered loudly and the lights went out. (3) The coach took the microphone to announce the contest winners.**
3. Generalizes knowledge and understanding of human characteristics, interactions, concepts, and ideas to new situations.	SLP: **From what you know about young girls having fun, what do you think Goldilocks would have done if the bears had not come home?** S: **She would have run home, gathered her friends, and led them to the bears' charming little cottage.**
4. Describes or takes various perspectives to view a situation.	SLP: **Imagine this story from two characters' viewpoints. First take the part of Goldilocks. Then take the part of Baby Bear. How were your feelings different when playing the two characters?** S: **When I was Goldilocks, I felt curious and adventurous. When I was Baby Bear, I was angry and frightened when I walked into our house.**
5. Imagines and predicts numerous possibilities ("What if ______?").	SLP: **What if your mom were the principal of this school? How would school be different for you?** S: Several students contrast their perspectives.

(continues)

Objectives	Examples
6. Summarizes complex stories, novels, plays, and oral or written reports.	SLP: **Summarize the story. Include the main character, setting, plot, and resolution.** S: **This novel is about Isabella, a 13-year-old girl who . . .**
7. Summarizes issues, opinions, and points of view of oneself and others gathered from various sources.	SLP: **We have heard the debate. Summarize each debater's opinion and point of view.** S: Writes a list of the debaters, with a few sentences by each that describe their opinions and points of view.
8. Supports and evaluates opinions of a text with facts and details.	SLP: **Each of you has a different point of view about what led to Romeo's and Juliet's deaths. Write a paragraph to support your opinion.** S: Students debate and write their opinions.
Short-Term Goal: Applies and evaluates ideas in hypothetical situations by supporting opinions and critiquing	
9. Evaluates the content and form of own performance.	SLP: **After you solve a problem, what questions could you ask yourself to evaluate your performance?** S: **How successful was my solution? What did I learn from the situation? What would I do in a similar difficult experience?**
10. Evaluates and chooses strategies for attacking problems and interpreting content.	SLP: **Your assignment is to prepare a speech about a prominent citizen. What strategies will you use to attack the assignment?** S: **I will ask for an appointment to interview our mayor and ask these questions: What do you like best about your work? What is the hardest part? What makes you proudest of our city?**
11. Explores the consequences of choices and decisions prior to and during the act of deciding.	SLP: **Let's talk about the ways you use free time during this class. Think about the consequences of your choices and decisions for the best use of the time.** S: **I'll list the consequences of using the time to study versus to daydream.**
12. Evaluates and chooses strategies for completing assignments, such as study groups, outlines, and visual organizers. (See Appendix C.)	SLP: **When preparing for your test, think about and select strategies for remembering information.** S: **I will ask myself which strategy will be best for me. For this test I will use visual organizers because at this point I need to organize my ideas. Then I'll study with a group.**

Thinking About Your Own Thinking

Yearly Goal: *To think about one's own thinking (metacognition) in order to make decisions and solve problems*

Objectives	Examples
1. Recognizes when a situation is being perceived flexibly or rigidly by self and/or others.	SLP: **Tell your partner the steps in your plan for your project. Try to recognize the flexibility or rigidity in your own thinking and in your partner's. Afterward, write down your own thinking.** S: (writes) Mia seemed defensive. I don't understand. I think I may be resisting her feedback, too. I will keep on listening. She has good ideas.
2. Delays making judgments about information by recognizing the need to allow patterns time to emerge.	SLP: **As you gather information about types of whales, you will notice patterns beginning to emerge. Become aware of your thinking, and notice what emerges.** S: This is my thinking. I want to get this report on types of whales finished quickly. However, as I've read about these amazing creatures, I find myself wanting to write about whale conservation instead. I'll find a good source so I can write about helping whales survive.
3. Expresses the joy of thinking by consciously exploring, designing, and playing with ideas.	SLP: **Notice your thoughts as you and your partners plan your presentation. What surprising ideas come as you play with ideas? Try brainstorming and see what bubbles up. Remember, there are no wrong answers.** S: My partner and I are asking ourselves "What would happen if . . . ?" questions. Thinking is fun!
4. Observes the "think aloud" process modeled by a teacher.	SLP: **I will model the "think aloud" process as I read the story aloud. Later I'll ask you to join me in thinking aloud. "Summer is the best time on the Island of the Blue Dolphins."** SLP: **I am thinking: This story will happen on an island. Why is summer the best time on the island? Now you join me in the think-aloud.** S: This story makes me think of when I visited an island with my family. The water was deep blue. It's easy to imagine the island in this story.

(continues)

Objectives	Examples
5. Describes own thinking while problem solving.	SLP: **Think aloud as you figure out the meaning of the word *decomposed* in the sentence "As the paper pulp decomposed, bad smells welled up from the Nashua River."** S: **I am thinking *composed* of is about parts that make up something. So *decomposed* could mean that the parts disintegrate or decompose or rot. As the pulp rotted along with all the trash, it polluted the river.**
6. Poses own study questions to use while preparing for a test.	SLP: **Write your own study questions to prepare for next week's test. Remember past tests to help you imagine the upcoming test questions.** S: **Since I've had two tests in Mr. Jones's history class, I know his pattern. I think he will ask questions like these: Why was it hard to travel from one place to another in colonial times? How did people in the colonies get news?**
7. Noncritically observes and describes the thinking of others.	SLP: **Read a biography of a person who has achieved dramatic recognition. Describe the person's thinking processes without judging him or her.** S: **I learned that Mary Lou Retton is the first woman outside Eastern Europe to win the Olympic all-around title. Retton may have thought, "I was born with athletic talent. I want to be the best athlete I can be. I'll train hard. I'll think encouraging thoughts."**
8. Shows awareness of and clarifies own thinking terminology.	SLP: **As you watch the video about student conflict, listen for high-intensity words or generalized terminology. Clarify the words and explain your thinking.** S: **I heard the sentence "They always do it." I think to myself, "Who is *they*? What does *always* mean?"**
9. Looks for alternatives when a solution doesn't work during a building project.	SLP: **Let's imagine how to reconstruct a block tower that fell down. Think about reasons the block tower fell, and choose a different way to build it.** S: **I think the base was too narrow. It needs to be wider and stronger.**
10. Considers alternative ways to gather written information when the first sources were not adequate.	SLP: **You are having difficulty finding information you need about Mark Twain's childhood. Describe your thinking about alternative solutions.** S: **I'll reconsider my strategy to look in the library for information because I'm not finding enough about his childhood. I'll search the Internet to find out about Twain's childhood.**

Unit 5

Organization and Study Skills

Organization and study skills are used across the spectrum of daily activities that involve planning and completing tasks. A variety of activities require these skills, from planning a social schedule and cooking from a recipe to planning and carrying out a shopping trip. Organization and study skills are vital to curriculum tasks in listening, speaking, reading, and writing. Skills include organizing notes into a written report, planning and carrying out a project over several days, and planning the steps of a science experiment. The skills in this area support any assigned school activities that involve planning for the timely and appropriate completion of tasks.

There are many students with weak organization and study skills, among both students with language disorders and those not affected by such difficulties. Organization and study skills are often especially deficient in students with language impairments, executive function disorders, and attention-deficit disorders. Students with Asperger's syndrome struggle with schedule and time management. As educational, vocational, and social expectations increase with age, the effects of these deficiencies become increasingly negative.

Students who have acquired strong organization and study skills have discovered an important truth: It's their responsibility to learn. They have discovered that they are the ones who must make learning occur—it doesn't just happen. Students with language and learning disorders can make this discovery. Direct instruction in organization and study skills improves these important skills and provides students with a key to learning.

The objectives in this unit are designed to be adapted for students with special needs, such as those with Asperger's syndrome or executive function disorders. Students with executive function disorders have difficulty with complex tasks, such as attention, inhibition, planning, organizing, and working memory (Nelson, 2010). Transitions and scheduling are especially difficult for students with these disorders. These students will benefit from visual supports when implementing the objectives. Schedules and calendars are especially helpful because they alert the student to changes in routines and help the student develop a richer concept of time. Kowalski (2002) suggested that visual schedules be made discrete by putting them on bookmarks to help students avoid being rejected as different. Because teacher expectations and student abilities vary, it is important to consult with classroom teachers to verify the grade-level and ability-level expectations for the student.

Description of Contents

The objectives in this unit are especially designed for students who may be seen by speech–language pathologists (SLPs), but they are applicable to any students who need to improve their ability to gather and evaluate information and organize their own tasks, time, space, materials, and attitude. Students with disabilities are not likely to acquire these abilities without help. Direct instruction, however, will lead to improvement and support academic success. This unit of Organization and Study Skills is divided into four areas with these short-term objectives.

Organizes and Manages Tasks, Time, and Study Schedules. The objectives in this section focus on helping students plan ahead so that they can complete tasks on time. Students are guided to analyze tasks so that they can anticipate any difficulties and materials they will need.

Organizes and Manages Study Space and Materials. This section has objectives for a basic requirement for studying well. The ability to organize one's study materials and study space is crucial to study skills both at home and at school. Included here are objectives for using a planner or assignment book, a skill that requires guidance to be mastered by students with special needs.

Manages Classroom Attitude for School Success. These objectives focus on what students need to do to make the most of their classroom learning time. Using polite words when talking with the teacher and taking responsibility for their own mistakes indicate that students are taking learning seriously. Managing one's attitude toward learning is a step toward being a responsible student.

Acquires Study Skills to Gather and Manage Information. These objectives target skills that students need to acquire information from books and other information sources. These skills span a variety of abilities. The objectives begin with skills young students can learn, such as skimming and highlighting information. For older students and students with more advanced skills, the objectives extend to taking efficient notes and locating information from a variety of sources.

Organization and Study Skills

Yearly Goal: *To organize and manage tasks, time, space, materials, and study schedules; show positive attitudes toward school; and effectively use, gather, and manage information*

Objectives	Examples
Short-Term Goal: Organizes and manages tasks, time, and study schedules	
1. Plans ahead before beginning a project.	SLP: **It's important to plan ahead for projects. Let's talk about the science project that is due next week. (1) What materials will you need? (2) What do you think they will cost? (3) Where can you get them?**
2. Analyzes tasks and anticipates difficulties related to, and needs for, information.	SLP: **Your group in theater class is getting ready to present a play. What do you think you need to do to get started? Is there anything that might be difficult?** S: **Yes, one of the characters in our play is a doctor. That character will need a stethoscope. We need to think about where to find one.**
3. Follows logical steps to complete assignments.	SLP: **You have been assigned to write a history report on Marie Curie. Tell me what steps you will take.** S: **First, I'll look for information on her childhood. Next, I will learn more about her career, and then I'll find out about her Nobel Prizes. I'll keep track of the authors of my sources of information.**
4. Prioritizes tasks required to complete several assignments.	SLP: **I know this is a really busy week for you. How can you work on all of your school assignments?** S: **I think I will list the assignments by importance and complete them one at a time.**
5. Completes tasks on time.	SLP: **How can you be sure that you get all of your schoolwork finished on time?** S: **I will keep a calendar and write down each assignment and the day it is due. Then I will put a check mark by each one when I finish it and turn it in.**
Short-Term Goal: Organizes and manages study space and materials	
6. Organizes study materials at school.	SLP: **Organization at school will save you a lot of time and stress. It's so helpful to know where everything is. Let's look at your locker and your desk area to see if we can think of better ways to organize your materials.** S: With help from the SLP, organizes textbooks, notebooks, files, backpack, assignment book, and locker.

(continues)

Objectives	Examples
7. Uses an assignment book.	SLP: **This week, I want you to keep this assignment book open on your desk. Each day, write down assignments as soon as the teacher gives them and write *none* if there is no homework. Bring it back next week, and we will talk about it.** S: Keeps assignment book and discusses its usefulness and any problems or new ways to use it with the SLP.
8. Plans a special, well-lighted study space at home with places for assignment book, textbooks, notebooks, folders, pencils, ruler, markers, and other things, such as a clock, a lamp, and a snack.	SLP: **It will be much easier to keep up with materials and complete your homework if you have a special study space at home. Talk about this with your family. Also think about if you seem to study best in your room, the kitchen, or away from the TV. Let me know next week about your home study space.** S: **My family and I chose the kitchen table as the best place for me to study. We cleaned off a shelf in a cabinet in the kitchen where I can keep all of the materials I need to study.**
Short-Term Goal: Manages classroom attitude for school success	
9. Pays attention to the teacher's voice and shows interest by nodding, keeping good eye contact, and so on.	SLP: **Paying attention to the teacher is important to be successful at school. What are some things you can do to help yourself pay attention?** S: **I can look at him when he is trying to get the students' attention, nod or react to what he is saying to show interest, and remember that it's my turn to listen.**
10. Shows polite behavior to the teacher.	SLP: **How can you be polite when asking for or receiving help from your teacher?** S: **I can wait patiently for my turn and remember to say "please" and "thank you."**
11. Asks questions to show interest.	SLP: **How can you show someone speaking to your class that you are interested?** S: **I can listen quietly, make eye contact, take notes if appropriate, and ask on-topic questions.**
12. Takes responsibility for own mistakes.	SLP: **Everyone makes mistakes. It's important for you to take responsibility and not to blame someone else. What could you say to your teacher if you forgot to bring your homework?** S: **I'm sorry. I left my essay at home because I didn't put it in my notebook.**

Objectives	Examples
Short-Term Goal: Acquires study skills to gather and manage information	
13. Skims books to preview and review written material.	SLP: **Sometimes you need to skim a book or a paragraph to decide if reading the whole thing will help you as you gather information for a report or project. Tell me some things you can do to skim the material.** S: **For a book, I could read the title and any reviews or summaries on the front and back cover. I could look at the titles of the chapters. For a paragraph, I can read the first and last sentences and notice dates and numbers to find answers to written questions for factual information.**
14. Underlines or highlights written material.	SLP: **It's often helpful to underline or highlight information when studying a book or class notes. Try to highlight only the key words or phrases. Look at this paragraph and show me what you would underline.** S: **The *Summer Olympics* take place every 4 years. They begin with an *Opening Ceremony* that features a Parade of Athletes who will compete in the games. They light the *Olympic Torch*. Athletes from all over the world gather for *17 days* to compete in many sports, including swimming, gymnastics, volleyball, soccer, and track and field. The athletes and teams placing first, second, or third win a *gold*, *silver*, or *bronze medal*, respectively.**
15. Takes notes efficiently.	SLP: **When you are taking notes in class, it's impossible to write down every word the teacher says. You should write down only the most important words and also learn some codes to be able to write faster. Here are some examples. You tell me what they mean: (1) b/c (2) = (3) re:** S: **(1) because (2) equals (3) regarding or about**
16. Uses writing as a study tool to clarify and remember information. (Refer to the visual organizers in Appendix C.)	SLP: **Create a visual organizer to help you sort the information for your book report. How could you visually organize the sequence of events in the book?** S: **I could make a timeline for entering important dates and events in the story along the line. Then I could connect each date to a rectangular box big enough to summarize the event.**

(continues)

Objectives	Examples
17. Surveys books and Internet to locate information.	SLP: **There is so much information available in books and on the Internet that it can be overwhelming. What are some good ways to locate the information you need?** S: **If I need information for a school assignment, I can scan tables of contents, chapter titles, graphics, and pictures in books and on the Internet. That will help me save time in choosing sources for my report.**
18. Evaluates the credibility of information resources, including how the writer's motivation may affect credibility.	SLP: **Just because you read something in a book or on the Internet, you should not assume that it is true or correct. What can you do to see if it is credible information?** S: **I can see who wrote it, when it was written, and why the author wrote it. That will help me make an informed decision on whether it is true and reliable.**

Unit 6

Listening

Functional Auditory Processing

- Auditory Discrimination
- Auditory Figure Ground
- Auditory Memory

Following Spoken Instructions

- Listening in Different Situations
- Listening With Empathy and Understanding
- Listening to Comprehend Information
- Listening to Evaluate a Message

The importance of listening in the life of students is impossible to overestimate. Listening is the most basic communication skill. It is the basis of speaking, reading, and writing. Its careful development is crucial to success in relationships with other people. Students' school success is dependent on adequate listening skills. The demands on listening abilities of students have never been greater. Parents, teachers, and speakers throughout the media demand the attention of students in the everyday world of school and home.

The term *listening* can mean many things. Different terminology is used in professional literature to describe problems with listening in individuals with normal hearing acuity. The term *auditory processing* has been used since the 1950s, when it was first introduced by Myklebust (1954). Since then, meaning for the term has gone through many changes. Richard (2001) summarized the influence of clinical and scientific research since 1954 that gradually resulted in the differentiation into two areas of what has been called auditory processing. These areas are *central auditory processing* and *language processing*. In this context, the term *processing* refers to a neurological activity, a "moving back and forth between auditory features of the signal and language features of meaning" (Richard, 2001, p. 18). The term *central auditory processing* applies when hearing acuity is normal but there are problems interpreting acoustic signals, such as pitch, loudness, and temporal aspects. Specifically, central auditory processing refers to listening difficulties related to the central auditory nervous system. An auditory processing disorder is a "deficit in the perceptual processing of auditory information in the central nervous system" (Bellis, 2004, p. 22) and includes poor auditory performance for basic auditory behaviors, such as the temporal aspects of audition and performing with competing or degraded acoustic signals. "Symptoms of auditory processing disorder overlap with those of other learning and attentional difficulties, making it challenging to accurately diagnose this disorder. Symptoms include difficulty paying attention, poor listening skills, difficulty following multistep directions, slow processing time, and impaired language and literacy development" (American Speech-Language-Hearing Association, 2005).

The term *language processing* is the second area of auditory processing. Specifically, language processing refers to listening deficits related to cortical structures above the brain stem, focusing primarily on left temporal lobe language functions. This term applies to not understanding the meaning of an acoustic signal although it was heard accurately. It is a problem with "the ability to use the linguistic code to attach meaning to the acoustic signal" (Richard, 2004, p. 7). Most problems with listening among school students are probably at the level of interpreting spoken messages (Richard, 2001).

The terms *central auditory processing* and *language processing* are helpful in designing therapy. Their distinction contributed to the organization of this unit. Because of advances and changes in the field, many activities that were formerly designed to improve auditory processing are now referred to as *phonological awareness* activities. This book provides numerous objectives for phonological awareness in Literacy: Reading, which has objectives for rhyming, phoneme identification, auditory closure, sound deletion and substitution, and sound blending.

Description of Contents

The organization of the objectives in this unit is derived from the two aspects of listening: auditory processing and language processing. Functional Auditory Processing focuses on skills that rely on both auditory processing and language processing. Listening in Different Situations focuses on objectives for language processing or understanding higher levels of information.

Functional Auditory Processing. This section provides objectives for auditory discrimination (beginning with discrimination of differences in loudness, pitch, and tone), auditory figure–ground (listening in the presence of background noise), auditory memory (using information stored in short-term memory), and following spoken instructions.

Listening in Different Situations. This section provides objectives to help students listen on a variety of levels, such as empathic listening and critical listening. Listening goals include listening with empathy while helping friends solve problems, listening for comprehension, and listening critically to judge message validity.

Auditory Discrimination

Yearly Goal: *To distinguish between sounds that are acoustically similar, including environmental sounds, pitch, volume, phonemes, and words*

CCSS.ELA-LITERACY.RF.K.2 and RF.1.2
CCSS.ELA-LITERACY.RF.K.2.A
CCSS.ELA-LITERACY.RF.K.2.D and RF.1.2.C
CCSS.ELA-LITERACY.RF.K.2.E

Objectives	Examples
Short-Term Goal: Discriminates differences in loudness, pitch, and tone	
1. Listens and tells the differences in loudness between nonverbal sounds, such as a door slamming and a pencil dropping.	SLP: **I'm going to make some sounds. If the sound is loud, cover your ears. If it's soft, put your finger to your lips.**
2. Discriminates differences between low- and high-pitched notes.	SLP: **Listen while I play this recording of different instruments and voices. Point down when a low tone is heard and point up when a high tone is heard.**
3. Discriminates differences in loudness of various vocal tones.	SLP: **I am going to use my voice in different ways. Is this loud or soft? (1) whispers, (2) sings a lullaby, (3) yells to someone in another room.** S: **(1) soft, (2) soft, (3) loud**
Short-Term Goal: Associates a sound with its source	
4. Identifies animal sounds and matches them to toy animals.	SLP: **Let's play with this toy barn and animals. I am going to make some animal sounds. When you hear an animal's sound, put that animal in the barn.** S: Hears sound of a cow and puts the cow in the barn.
5. Listens to environmental sounds and points to the pictures that represent the sounds heard.	SLP: **Look at this picture scene and listen to these recorded sounds. Point to the pictures that go with each sound.** S: Hears a train whistle and points to the train.
Short-Term Goal: Discriminates differences in phonemes and in words	
6. Tells whether two spoken words are the same or different.	SLP: **Listen to me say two words. If they are the same, show me a thumbs up. If they are different, show me a thumbs down: (1) *bake, take*; (2) *bus, bus*.** S: (1) thumbs down, (2) thumbs up
7. Picks out the common consonant spoken in a group of several words.	SLP: **Listen to my words: *peach, pear, plum, prune*. What sound do you hear in the beginning of all of them?** S: **/p/**

(continues)

Objectives	Examples
8. Picks out the common vowel spoken in a group of different words.	SLP: **While we are talking about body parts, listen to these vocabulary words: *heel, see, breathe, knee*. What vowel sound do you hear?** S: /i/
9. Identifies beginning sounds in words as same or different.	SLP: **Listen to these words from our story today. If they start with the same sound, hold up the happy face picture. If they start with different sounds, hold up the sad face: (1) *mouse, milk;* (2) *comb, nap*.** S: (holds up) (1) happy face, (2) sad face
10. Identifies ending sounds in words as same or different.	SLP: **The last car in a train is a caboose. Hold this caboose and listen to my two words. If they have the same last sound, put the caboose on the train. If the last sounds are different, we will leave the caboose off. Here are the words: (1) *hat, ham;* (2) *phone, man*.** S: (1) Does not put the caboose on the train. (2) Puts the caboose on the train.
11. Identifies two rhyming words from a spoken list.	SLP: **I am going to read a list of words while we walk around in a circle. When you hear two words that rhyme, sit down. Listen: *horse, cow, pig, big*.** S: Sits down upon hearing the rhyming words *pig, big*.
12. Identifies the beginning, middle, or ending consonant of a spoken word and changes it to make a new word.	SLP: **Listen to this word: *ticket*. Tell me the consonant sound at the beginning, middle, and end.** S: **beginning /t/, middle /k/, end /t/**
13. Listens to directions to change one sound in a word to make a new word.	SLP: **Choose an animal from the barn and listen as I say its name: *pig*. What is the first sound in *pig*? What new words can you make if you change that first sound?** S: **The first sound is /p/. I can think of the words *dig, big, jig, rig,* and *wig*.**
14. Identifies the vowel in a spoken word and changes it to make a new word.	SLP: **What vowel sound do you hear in the word *beet*? Change the vowel sound to make new words. For each word that you say, stack a block to build a tower.** S: (stacks a block on his tower each time he says a new word) **/i/ is the vowel in *beet*. The new words I can think of are *bait, boat, bat, bite,* and *bought*.**
15. Listens to a story and counts how often a target phoneme occurs.	SLP: **Listen to this paragraph. Count the number of times you hear the /s/ sound.**

Auditory Figure–Ground

Yearly Goal: *To demonstrate the ability to differentiate a primary auditory stimulus from other background auditory stimuli*

Objectives	Examples
Short-Term Goal: Localizes sounds in the environment	
1. Locates a given or named sound in the environment. ("Find the ticking clock.")	SLP: **Let's play a hide-and-seek game. Can you find the music playing? Now listen and look for the ticking clock.**
2. Points to or turns the body in the direction of a noise or voice heard while eyes are closed.	SLP: **Close your eyes and listen for my voice. When you hear me say your name, keep your eyes closed and point to where you think I am.**
3. Identifies common environmental sounds in the room (air ducts, computers, fans).	SLP: **We are going to walk around the school, inside and outside. When we stop, I will ask you what sounds you hear.** S: Listens and identifies common sounds. **I hear a bell ringing, the hall clock ticking, and a car horn.**
Short-Term Goal: Listens in the presence of distracting sounds	
4. Recognizes words spoken one at a time in the presence of a recording of static or white noise playing in the room.	SLP: **Sometimes there is noise in the background, and it makes it hard to listen to the teacher. I am going to play a recording of a noise called static or white noise, then I will say some words. Listen carefully and say each word after me: *window, horse, playground.***
5. Follows simple directions or answers questions spoken in the presence of static or white noise.	SLP: **While this static or white noise plays in the background, I want you to listen carefully and follow my directions. Put the red block on top of two blue blocks, and so on.**
6. Participates successfully in an auditory listening task with instrumental music in the background.	SLP: **I am going to play some pretty music while I read this story to you. Keep listening carefully to the story, and be ready to answer my questions.** S: Listens to the story and answers the questions.
7. Completes a spoken instruction activity while a story is being read in the background.	SLP: **I am going to play a recording of someone reading a story. At the same time, I am going to tell you what to do on your work sheet. Try to ignore the story and pay attention only to my voice. Here is your first direction: Color the rectangle blue.**

(*continues*)

Objectives	Examples
8. Identifies possible interfering distracting noises in the classroom and compensates by changing her work location in the room.	SLP: **Are there some noisy places in your classroom that make it hard for you to concentrate on what the teacher is saying? Where are they, and what could you do to make it easier for you to listen?** S: **My desk is by the door. The noise in the hallway makes it hard for me to listen to the teacher. I could tell him about it and ask to move to another part of the room.**

Auditory Memory

Yearly Goal: *To increase auditory memory for information, including contextual and rote academic sequences, such as counting and poems*

Objectives	Examples
Short-Term Goal: Remembers sequences in the order named	
1. Remembers and picks up two objects named.	SLP: **Look at the toys on our table. Pick up the ones that I say. Pick up the block and the car.**
2. Points to shapes in the order named.	SLP: **I drew some shapes on the board. Let's name all of the shapes. Now go to the board and point to the circle and then the triangle.** S: Points to the circle and then to the triangle.
3. Repeats a series of people's names.	SLP: **Listen as I say the names of some of your classmates: Raul, Grace, and Brayden. Now say them back to me in the same order.**
4. Repeats a series of animal sounds in sequence to help tell a story.	SLP: **Help me tell this story. Listen for the animal sounds and say them back in the same order I say them: *woof, baa, cluck, oink*.**
5. Repeats various nonverbal sound patterns.	SLP: **Let's play Listen to the Leader. I want you to tap the same pattern I tap.** Tap, tap, pause, tap, tap, tap. S: Repeats pattern by tapping on the table.
6. Remembers and repeats rote sequences within their context (poems, rhymes).	SLP: **Listen and watch as I say and act out the poem "Twinkle, Twinkle, Little Star." Say each line after me. Now let's say the whole poem together.**
7. Remembers and repeats rote academic sequences (days of the week, counting, alphabet).	SLP: **It's Calendar Time! Let's say the days of the week together while I point to the calendar.**
8. Repeats phone numbers and addresses of people, businesses, and residences familiar to the student.	SLP: **Phone numbers and addresses are important things to remember. I'm going to say your mom's phone number, and you can say it back to me.**

Objectives	Examples
Short-Term Goal: Remembers identified words, multiple items, details, and messages	
9. Recalls details and answers basic fact questions about a spoken sentence.	SLP: **Listen carefully to my sentence and be ready to answer a question about it. John ran down the road. Who ran down the road?** S: **John**
10. Remembers an identified word and signals when it occurs during a story read aloud.	SLP: **Let's jump! Now listen to my story and raise your hand every time you hear the word *jump*.** S: Raises hand when he hears the word *jump*.
11. Remembers and repeats as many related words as possible from a spoken list.	SLP: **We have been learning about kinds of birds. I'm going to name some birds, and I want you to repeat as many as you can remember. Listen: robin, cardinal, sparrow, eagle, seagull, dove, wren, blue jay, parrot.** S: Names as many birds as she can remember.
12. Identifies missing items from an orally presented list.	SLP: **Listen to my directions for our project. We'll need magazines, scissors, tape, paper, and markers. I said we'll need magazines, tape, and markers. What did I forget?** S: **Scissors and paper**
13. Recalls and repeats a phone message.	SLP: **I am going to pretend to call you on the phone. I want you to remember my message and tell it to your classmate. Here is the message: Tell Shirley that I want her to bring something for show-and-tell and a snack to school tomorrow.** S: Tells classmate the correct message.
14. Retells a joke or a story told by someone else.	SLP: **I am going to tell you a funny joke. Listen carefully, and then tell the same joke to your classmate.** S: Tells the joke to a classmate.
15. Recalls and describes past events or personal experiences.	SLP: **Abby, we missed you on the field trip last week. Robyn, tell Abby five things that you remember from the field trip.** S: **We rode on a bus and went to the country. We saw bluebonnets and a creek. We had a picnic lunch.**

Following Spoken Instructions

Yearly Goal: *To understand, sequence, and follow a variety of spoken instructions*

Objectives	Examples
1. Imitates and follows spoken instructions that require body movement.	SLP: **We are going to play Follow the Leader. Watch and listen and do what I say. Hop on one foot.**
2. Follows one-step commands when given visual cues. (Speaker gestures with hand and says, "Come here.")	SLP: **When your teacher tells you to do something, also watch for a gesture that will help you understand the direction. Let's try some. (1)** Gestures with hand: **Come here. (2)** Points to table: **Put your paper here.** S: Follows commands correctly.
3. Follows one-step motor commands.	SLP: **We are going to play Simon Says. If I say Simon Says to do something, it's your turn to do it. Let's try one: Simon Says touch your toes.** S: Does what Simon says.
4. Follows two-step motor commands in the order given.	SLP: **I'm going to tell you two things to do. Then it will be your turn to do them in the right order. Listen: Sit down and raise your hand.** S: Follows directions in the correct order.
5. Follows three-step motor commands in the order given.	SLP: **Let's see if you can remember three things to do in the correct order. Listen: Stand up, turn around, wave your hand.** S: Listens then follows three directions in the correct order.
6. Follows directions that require an understanding about the location of an object.	SLP: **Listen for my directions that tell you where to find or put something. Bring me the book on the bottom shelf.**
7. Follows commands presented in *if . . . then* form.	SLP: **We are going to talk about following directions that have the words *if . . . then*. Listen to the whole direction. If you are finished with your spelling paper, then you may choose a book to read. Tell me what that means.** S: **It means that I can read a book only if I finish my spelling paper.**
8. Follows commands that involve the concepts of left and right.	SLP: **Show me your right hand. Now show me your left hand. Let's sing and dance to the "Hokey Pokey."** S: Follows directions such as "put your right hand in or put your left foot out."

Objectives	Examples
9. Follows locational directions that require paper-and-pencil responses.	SLP: **Listen carefully for where I tell you to draw on this work sheet. Draw a line under the bear. Draw a circle next to the tree.**
10. Follows commands that involve time concepts.	SLP: **Be sure to listen to when you should do things in my instructions. Before you begin the experiment, put on the safety glasses.** S: Follows directions in correct order.
11. Follows spoken instructions that involve comparatives and superlatives.	SLP: **Listen for some special words in my instructions that will tell you exactly what to do on your work sheet. Put an X on the largest animal. Circle the ball that is smaller.** S: Puts an X on the elephant and circles the golf ball.
12. Follows spoken instructions that involve opposites.	SLP: **This is a funny game about opposites. Do the opposite of what I say: smile.** S: Frowns
13. Gives an oral message correctly to another person after hearing the message.	SLP: **We are going to play the Telephone Game. Listen while I tell you something. Then tell the same message to your classmate.**

Listening With Empathy and Understanding

Yearly Goal: *To develop abilities to show empathy and understanding when listening to friends*

Objectives	Examples
1. Shows empathy by recognizing a friend's feelings during a conversation.	SLP: **When having a conversation with your friend, how could you show that you recognize her feelings?** S: **If she is happy or excited, I can smile and use a happy tone of voice. If she is sad, I might put my hand on her shoulder and show with my face that I also feel sad for her.**
2. Keeps a friend's point of view in mind when listening to the friend's problem.	SLP: **Let's pretend that your friend is telling you about a problem, such as not making the baseball team. When you listen to him, it's important to think about his point of view. What could that be?** S: **I might think it's not that important, but I need to remember that he has been practicing for a long time and really wanted to make the team.**
3. Responds with words and actions to what a friend is saying.	SLP: **How can you show your friend that you are really listening to what he is saying?** S: **I could nod my head, lean toward him, and ask thoughtful questions.**

(continues)

Objectives	Examples
4. Resists judging and showing disapproval when a friend describes her own behavior.	SLP: **For you to be a good listener, it is important not to judge your friend. Suppose your friend told you that he skipped going to school one day and then got caught. What are some things you should not say to him?** S: **I would try not to say things like "I told you so" or "I can't believe you did that."**
5. Lets friends know that their feelings are acceptable.	SLP: **How could you show your friend that what he is feeling, such as sadness or nervousness or fear, is okay?** S: **I could show acceptance through caring facial expressions, posture, and tone of voice.**
6. Lets friends talk through their problems instead of giving quick solutions.	SLP: **Instead of giving a quick solution, tell me some things you could say that could help a friend solve a problem instead of trying to solve the problem for her.** S: **I could say things like "What do you think you should do?" or "Maybe it would help to talk to your teacher."**

Listening to Comprehend Information

Yearly Goal: *To develop abilities to listen responsibly in order to understand and recall information*

Objectives	Examples
1. Shows responsibility for listening for information about tasks, assignments, and instructions.	SLP: **In the classroom, you need to know when the teacher will give important information. What does your teacher do before she gives instructions?** S: **My teacher says things like "Listen" and "Eyes on me," or she turns the lights off and on.**
2. Increases ability to concentrate on the situation.	SLP: **Sometimes it's hard to listen to what you should. What could you do to help yourself concentrate on the speaker?** S: **I could sit closer to the speaker, take notes, make eye contact, and remove any objects that are distracting me.**
3. Uses all five senses to increase memory for what was heard.	SLP: **What are your five senses? How can you use them to help remember what you hear?** S: **Hearing: Listen carefully to the speaker. Seeing: Make eye contact with the speaker. Touching: Take notes or touch examples that are available. Smelling: Notice and remember any good aromas or unpleasant odors. Tasting: If food is involved, remember how things taste.**

Objectives	Examples
4. Selects the important parts of information to listen for.	SLP: **Sometimes there is just too much to remember. How can you decide the important parts to listen for?** S: **I will listen for the information that applies to me. I will listen for verbs that tell me what to do and nouns that tell me the materials I need.**
5. Asks questions when confused about a person's message.	SLP: **After listening carefully to a message, you might still be confused about it. How could you ask for more information? Give me an example.** S: **I could ask a question about specific parts of the information that I don't understand. I could say, "I'm sorry, but I don't know what a radiologist is. Could you explain that again?"**
6. Repeats the message as a strategy to confirm understanding.	SLP: **Repeating the message back to the person who just said it is a good way to be sure you understand and gives the speaker a chance to say "Right!" or "No, let me tell you again." Let's practice. I'll tell you all of the things that need to go home for homework tonight, and you can repeat them back to me.** S: Repeats back ***spelling book, red folder***, and math **paper.**

Listening to Evaluate a Message

Yearly Goal: *To develop abilities to evaluate a message before accepting or rejecting what was said*

CCSS.ELA-LITERACY.SL.K.2–SL.1.2
CCSS.ELA-LITERACY.SL.2.1.C
CCSS.ELA-LITERACY.SL.K.3–SL.3.3

Objectives	Examples
1. Thinks about information to decide if it is fact or opinion.	SLP: **How can we determine whether information that we read or hear is factual or merely one person's opinion? Why is it important to know?** S: **We can listen carefully but also ask ourselves if the information can be proved. Opinions are important, but there can be many different opinions on one topic. If it cannot be proved, we should not believe it as a fact.**

(continues)

Objectives	Examples
2. Picks out opinions that sound like facts.	SLP: **Listen to this commercial about breakfast cereal. Tell me which parts of the commercial are facts and which parts are opinions.** S: **Facts: This breakfast cereal has Vitamin B. It has almonds in it. Opinions: It will make us strong. It's the best thing you will ever eat.**
3. Judges the validity of information to decide whether it is dependable.	SLP: **Just because you hear something on TV does not make it true. How can you find out if the information is valid?** S: **I could find out if the speaker has a lot of experience in that area. I can listen to see if he tells where he got his facts. I can research the information on my own to see if I find the same conclusion.**
4. Listens to the whole message before deciding if it's dependable.	SLP: **Sometimes it's tempting to make up your mind about what someone is saying before you hear all of the message. Why should you listen to the whole thing?** S: **The speaker might add some facts or examples at the end of the message that would lead me to a different conclusion.**
5. Asks questions to aid in judging and clarifying a message.	SLP: **It's not wise to judge a message unless you understand it. What could you do to help yourself understand?** S: **I could ask the speaker to give examples or clarify any confusing statements.**
6. Allows others to respond to a speaker's message in different ways without putting them down.	SLP: **Several people can hear the same message and all feel differently about it. Some may agree, others might be angry, and others might not believe the speaker. What can you do to respect everyone's response?** S: **I can remember that people from other backgrounds and with other experiences may react differently to the same message. I should not put them down for their opinion but respect them for their ideas. It's okay if my friend's response is different from mine.**

Unit 7

Literacy: Reading

Learning to Read

- **Reading Readiness: Age 3 Months to Kindergarten**
- **Phonological Awareness: PreK–Grade 1**
- **Reading Accuracy: Grades 1–5**
- **Reading Fluency: Grades 1–12**

Reading to Learn

- **Reading Comprehension of Literature: Grades 1–3**
- **Reading Comprehension of Literature: Grades 4–8**
- **Reading Comprehension of Informational Text: Grades 4–8**

Most children learn to read somewhat quickly, but, unfortunately, learning to read is a challenge for a surprising number of children. Reading disability comprises up to 80% of students who receive special education instruction. Shaywitz (2005, p. 28) reported that some 20% of school-age children were reading below their age, grade, or level of ability. The National Research Council concluded in 1998 that the education of 25% to 40% of U.S. students was imperiled because of poor reading ability (Shaywitz, 2005, p. 30). Reading is the major avenue to learning. It is the key to success.

Speech–language pathologists (SLPs) play an important supportive role in planning the treatment and identification of reading disabilities. Children with language disorders are more likely to struggle with reading and spelling (Justice, 2010, p. 214). An area of particular difficulty diagnosed as an aspect of dyslexia is phonological awareness. Children with this diagnosis require early intervention if they are to become readers. It is critical to have participation of SLPs on the Individualized Education Program (IEP) team to plan intervention for students with reading disabilities (Justice, 2010, p. 138).

Reading is a complex cognitive, perceptual, and linguistic process that can be defined as the operations by which a person constructs meaning from printed symbols. Reading includes two general parts: *decoding* and *comprehension*. Decoding is the process the reader uses to transform print to words. Comprehension is the process by which one understands and interprets language. Decoding and comprehension are equally important. To decode without comprehension is not reading, just as attempting to comprehend without decoding is not reading. In the early grades (K–3), instructional goals in reading focus on *learning to read* (Snow, Scarborough, & Burns, 1999). In third grade, there is a shift from learning to read to *reading to learn*. The emphasis changes to comprehension in Grades 4–8 (Owens, 2016). The shift is reflected in the sequence of objectives in the Common Core State Standards and the objectives in this reading unit.

The Common Core State Standards grade levels were used to suggest grade levels for reading objectives in *The SLP's IEP Companion, Third Edition*. In this reading unit, for example, Grade 8 is the upper level for standards from the Common Core. If a child's IEP, however, recommends support in reading for a student in a grade higher than Grade 8, then the reading objectives in *The SLP's IEP Companion* will most likely be appropriate regardless of the student's grade level.

Many of the objectives in the reading unit correlate with standards in the Common Core. This unit has the largest number of applicable standards of any of the units in *The SLP's IEP Companion*. Some objectives in *The SLP's IEP Companion*, however, do not match a standard. We included these objectives because we have used them ourselves and found them to be effective in reading intervention. We think they will be helpful to you, too.

Description of Contents

This unit is organized in two parts: Learning to Read and Reading to Learn. In general, objectives for Learning to Read are suitable for the majority of younger children in Grades K–3, whereas objectives in Reading to Learn are designed for children and youth in Grades 4–12. The exception to this general division is the section Reading Fluency, which has objectives that apply to students in Grades 1–12. Reading Fluency Common Core objectives end at Grade 5; however, they continue to apply to students in any grade who need to improve reading fluency (reading quickly and accurately with good understanding).

Learning to Read

Reading Readiness: Age 3 Months to Kindergarten. The purpose of this section's objectives is to help students develop an early knowledge or acquaintance with books, pictures, and print awareness, such as knowing the direction in which print goes across a page. Print awareness comes through interaction between the child and the parents or caregivers (Owens, 2016, p. 343). These early literacy-readiness skills precede reading and specific sound awareness.

Phonological Awareness: PreK–Grade 1. Use these early literacy objectives to help children develop beginning awareness of sounds and syllables and the ability to manipulate them in spoken words. At this level, students learn skills in rhyming, sound and syllable identification, sound blending, and sound deletion and substitution.

Reading Accuracy: Grades 1–5. Common Core State Standards in this section will be appropriate for students in Grades 1–3 and can be extended to Grade 5 for some students with IEPs. The objectives are designed to help students apply decoding rules to words in order to increase their comfort level in reading. Students strengthen decoding skills for words, beginning with labels and CVC (consonant–vowel–consonant) words, and progressing to words with double vowels (*ea, oa, ai*), consonant clusters, prefixes, and suffixes; multisyllabic words; and irregularly spelled words.

Reading Fluency: Grades 1–12. Use this section to plan intervention for your students at any grade level who need to improve reading fluency. Children are generally comfortable with reading text when they can read about 19 out of 20 words correctly, or 95% (Justice, 2010, p. 278). Reading fluency supports reading comprehension. Fluent reading is the ability to read quickly and accurately with good understanding and with no need to sound out words part by part. Students must be able to read words accurately before they can read fluently. That is why some of the objectives are for word speed drills (Swigert, 2004), repeated oral reading (Calkins, 2001; Shaywitz, 2005), and independent reading level (the level at which a child reads with comfort) (Calkins, 2001).

Reading to Learn

Reading Comprehension of Literature: Grades 1–3. Use these objectives to plan lessons that help students read with understanding a variety of types of literature, such as poetry, stories, and textbooks. Unless children read with understanding, they are not reading.

Reading Comprehension of Literature: Grades 4–8. The purpose of these objectives is to guide students into reading, appreciating, and understanding various types of literature, such as fictional stories, myths, poetry, and novels. The objectives help lead students to higher thinking levels: reading with purpose; analyzing texts for their deeper meanings; making applications, inferences, and predictions; and developing new ideas.

Reading Comprehension of Informational Text: Grades 4–8. These students have learned to read but need to increase their reading comprehension. Use the objectives to help students understand and gain information from a variety of sources: written instructions, reference books, websites, and other factual texts, such as biographies and textbooks. The aim of these objectives is to help students improve their ability to read purposefully and to understand the underlying structure of a given text.

Description of Appendix C: Using Concept Maps as Visual Organizers for Reading and Writing

Appendix C provides examples of concept maps as visual organizers. The most basic concept map is the *simple causal narrative map*. Use it to help preschool students internalize a simple story structure as they learn to retell simple, one-episode stories.

Success with the simple causal narrative map can prepare for the use of the *story map* for emerging readers. At first, SLPs may want to ask the emerging reader to dictate the basic story while you write on the concept map. Later, children will create their own maps.

The *episode map* helps students analyze story parts and relate them to the whole. This map shows three episodes, but you can increase the number as needed. When your students begin to discover that each story episode in a multicausal story contains a problem (or complication) within the main story's main problem, they begin to approach reading with more curiosity and confidence. Their ability to understand complex relationships in stories increases.

The *compare-and-contrast map* is a flexible map with many uses. Students can use it to externalize their thoughts as they compare one story to another, one character to another, or a significant vocabulary word to another.

The *characterization map* is new to *The SLP's IEP Companion*. Use it to help your students understand and describe characters in stories by having them enter adjectives to describe a character. Use it during reading time or discussion afterward. It can also be used as a springboard for writing descriptions of characters.

Using concept maps as visual organizers relieves the burden on a student's auditory processing and memory abilities. That is because visual organizers help structure the child's thinking and bring the critical thinking process to a conscious level. Students can refer to the concept maps while engaged in thinking, organizing, and discussing what they have read. The process of making their own maps allows students with visual memory problems to store the conceptual maps of their mental models, provided the maps are not too complex. Thus, students construct an internal model that then helps them anticipate the structure of both literary and informational text. The improved comprehension not only increases knowledge but also builds confidence that extends into the next reading experience (Wiig & Wilson, 2001).

There are many resources for various types of visual organizers for reading, writing, and critical thinking. Among those are *Visual Tools for Constructing Knowledge* (Hyerle, 1996), *The Source for Dyslexia and Dysgraphia* (Richards, 1999), and *Map It Out: Visual Tools for Thinking, Organizing, and Communicating* (Wiig & Wilson, 2001). Students can also create their own concept maps. They can draw them or use computer programs. The user-friendly program *Inspiration 9.0* can be downloaded from the Internet. This resource allows students in Grades K–12 to create colorful concept maps and other visual organizers (Inspiration, 2016).

Reading Readiness: Age 3 Months to Kindergarten

Yearly Goal: *To develop the awareness of books, pictures, and print as early literacy skills that precede reading*

CCSS.ELA-LITERACY.RL.K.1 and RL.K.4
CCSS.ELA-LITERACY.RL.K.2
CCSS.ELA-LITERACY.RF.K.1, RF. K.1.A, RF. K.1.C, and RF. K.1.D
CCSS.ELA-LITERACY.RF.K.3.A
CCSS.ELA-LITERACY.RF.K.3.C

Objectives	Examples
Short-Term Goal: Develops awareness of books and pictures	
1. Shows awareness of books in various ways, such as mouthing, holding, dropping, and glancing at pictures.	SLP: **Let's play with these toys.** S: Chews the baby-safe book, bangs it on the table, or momentarily glances at some pictures.
2. Shows auditory and beginning visual and verbal interest in books.	SLP: **Let's read this book. The car says "beep-beep."** S: Listens, pats, or points to pictures and begins to imitate the teacher's picture-related noises, "beep-beep."
3. Names some objects or people in books.	SLP: **Let's look at this page. What is this?** S: **Car, bus, Mommy**
4. Shows beginning book orientation by holding the book right-side up and turning some pages.	SLP: **Look at all the books on our shelf. Choose your favorite book.** S: Holds the book right-side up and turns some pages.
5. Imitates some familiar actions pictured in books.	SLP: **Let's do what the animals in our book are doing.** S: Pretends to hop, sleep, and fly.
6. Pretends to read familiar picture books.	SLP: **Show me how you read your book.** S: Turns some pages in the book and pretends to read.
7. Protests if adult changes the story.	SLP: Leaves out or changes part of a familiar story. S: Protests with turning back to correct page: **No, not that.**
8. Participates in repeating familiar story lines or rhyming words from a book.	SLP: **Pretend you have something hard to do. Pretend to be the Little Engine That Could. While you work hard, whisper this with me: I think I can. I think I can.** S: Whispers "I think I can" while pretending to rake a pile of leaves.

Objectives	Examples
9. Uses phrases or short sentences to tell about a story.	SLP: **We get to look at *Clifford the Big Red Dog*. Tell me about this picture.** S: **Big dog. He is red. Clifford sleeping.**
10. Asks simple questions, such as "Who go?" or "What that?," about a book.	SLP: **Today we will read a new book.** Pauses for a question or asks child to imitate a question. S: **Who go? What that? Where dog?**
11. Predicts and anticipates parts of familiar stories.	SLP: Reads a book aloud. Before turning to the next page, asks, **What happens next?** S: **It's a butterfly!**
12. Shows responsibility in the use and care of books.	SLP: **You chose a book from the shelf. Tell me some ways to take care of our books.** S: **Keep it clean and dry. Don't write or color in it. Bring it back on time.**
13. Demonstrates an understanding of the language of books.	SLP: **Let's explore our new readers. Point to a letter, a word, the title, the front and back covers of the book, where we start to read, page 1, the next page, the top and bottom of the page, the first line, and the beginning and end of the sentence.** S: Points to the correct places in the book.
14. Retells familiar stories.	SLP: **Did you like *The Very Hungry Caterpillar*? I want you to retell the story in your own words.** S: Retells the story with prompting.
Short-Term Goal: Develops a beginning interest in print	
15. Recognizes and reads common signs and logos.	SLP: **Look at the sign in the picture. What does that *M* mean?** S: **McDonald's**
16. Recognizes own name in print.	SLP: **Good morning, Leonardo. Find your name on your locker and the jobs chart.** S: Puts belongings in the correct locker and points to his name on the jobs chart.
17. Finds letters in books that match the first letter in name.	SLP: **Point to the letter on this page that begins your first name.** S: Points to correct letter.
18. Points to and names familiar letters and makes some letter–sound matches.	SLP: **Point to some of the letters on this book cover. Name them and tell me what sounds they make.** S: Points to and names letters and makes correct associated sounds.
19. Tells if two printed letters are the same or different.	SLP: **Are these two letters the same or different?**

(*continues*)

Objectives	Examples
20. Matches uppercase and lowercase letters and names them correctly.	SLP: **Work with your partner to match these uppercase and lowercase letters and name them.** S: **Let's take turns matching the letters.**
21. Follows lines of text from left to right and top to bottom with finger.	SLP: **Point to the Papa Bear's words on this page while we say them together: Who has been sitting in my chair?**
22. Recognizes word boundaries.	SLP: **Point to each word on this page as I read it.**
23. Reads some common sight words.	SLP: **Read this word on the flash card. Now let's find it on this page in our book.** S: Reads the word *the* and then points to it in the book.

Phonological Awareness: PreK–Grade 1

Yearly Goal: *To increase awareness of sounds and syllables and the ability to manipulate them in spoken words as a part of reading readiness and early literacy*

CCSS.ELA-LITERACY.RF.K.2.A–RF.K.2.E
CCSS.ELA-LITERACY.RF.1.2.B–RF.1.2.D
CCSS.ELA-LITERACY.RF.1.2.C
CCSS.ELA-LITERACY.RF.1.2.D

Objectives	Examples
Short-Term Goal: Identifies or creates words that sound alike or rhyme: Rhyming	
1. Hears two words and determines if they rhyme.	SLP: **Do these words rhyme: *rack, back*? Yes. Now listen for more rhyming words. Hold up your happy face puppet when I say two words that rhyme. Hold up the sad face when two words do not rhyme: (1) *pop, top*; (2) *lip, lap*.** S: (1) Holds up happy face, (2) holds up sad face.
2. Names three objects or pictures and points to the two that rhyme.	SLP: **Name the three pictures on this page: *house, cat, mouse*. Circle the two pictures that rhyme. Then say the rhyming words.** S: Circles *house, mouse* while saying them.
3. Names three objects or pictures and points to the one that does not rhyme.	SLP: **Name the pictures on this page. Cross out the picture on each row that does not rhyme with the others.** S: Says **face, bag, race** and crosses out *bag*.
4. Completes the second line of a familiar poem with a rhyming word.	SLP: **Listen to this poem. Finish the poem with a rhyming word. Hickory Dickory Dock, the mouse ran up the _____.** S: **clock**

Objectives	Examples
5. Says a word that rhymes with an object or a picture.	SLP: **Say a word that rhymes with *nose*.** S: **Rose**
6. Names at least three words that rhyme with a given word.	SLP: **See how many words your group can come up with that rhyme with *bat*.** S: **Cat, fat, mat, rat, sat, tat**
Short-Term Goal: Identifies the number of syllables in a word and blends them into a word when they are given separately: Syllable identification and blending	
7. Tells how many syllables are heard in a spoken word.	SLP: **Do you like to eat fruit? Listen to the fruits I say. Clap your hands for each syllable in the name of the fruit I say: *strawberry*. How many times did you clap?** S: (claps three times) **three**
8. Thinks of a word with the same number of syllables as a given word.	SLP: **Let's name these food pictures. Say *apple*. Now think of another word with the same number of syllables.** S: **Lemon**
9. When given two choices of pictures and hears the name of one of the pictures spoken with segmented syllables, points to the correct picture.	SLP: **Did you like the story about wild animals? Look at these two pictures of a tiger and a lion. Circle the *ti-ger*.**
10. Says the correct word after hearing its segmented syllables.	SLP: **Guess what word I'm trying to say: *por-cu-pine*.** S: **Porcupine**
Short-Term Goal: Identifies the beginning sound in a word: Initial alliteration	
11. When looking at two pictures or objects, points to the one that starts with a given sound.	SLP: **We read about vehicles today. Point to the pictures of the vehicles that start with /b/.** S: Points to boat, bike.
12. When presented with three pictures or objects, points to two that start with the same sound.	SLP: **Listen as I name these pictures of musical instruments: *horn, harp, guitar*. Point to the two instruments that start with the same sound.** S: Points to horn, harp.
13. Says a word that starts with the same sound as a pictured word.	SLP: **Did you like the film about farm animals? Think of two words that start with the same sound as *chicken*.** S: **Children, cherry**
14. Says three words that begin with a given sound.	SLP: **Put your lips together and make a humming sound: *mmmm*. You said the sound of the letter *M*. Tell me three words that start with /m/.** S: **Moon, map, mom**

(*continues*)

Objectives	Examples
Short-Term Goal: Identifies the last sound in a word: Final alliteration	
15. When looking at two pictures or objects, points to the one that ends with a given sound.	SLP: **You are holding pictures of weather words. Stand up to show the picture that ends with /n/.** S: Stands up to show the picture of rain.
16. When presented with three pictures or objects, chooses the two that end with the same sound.	SLP: **Here are pictures of animal homes. Hold up the two animal home pictures that end with the same sound: *cave, nest, hive*.** S: Holds up and says **cave, hive**.
17. Says a word that ends with the same sound as a pictured word or object.	SLP: **Think of words that end with the same sounds. Tell me a word that ends with the same sound as *clap*.** S: **Top**
18. Thinks of three or more words that end with a given sound.	SLP: **See how many words you can think of that end with /p/.** S: **Cup, cap, mop, tape, ship, lip**
Short-Term Goal: Identifies whether a given sound occurs at the beginning, middle, or end of a word: Phoneme isolation	
19. Determines the position of a given sound in a pictured word.	SLP: **Listen carefully. Tell me if the /l/ sound comes at the beginning, middle, or end of this word: *log*.** S: **Beginning**
20. Pronounces the sound heard at the beginning, middle, or end of a word.	SLP: **What sound do you hear in the middle of the word *feet*? What sound is at the end?** S: **/i/, /t/**
Short-Term Goal: Blends and segments onsets and rimes of single-syllable spoken words: Onsets and rimes	
21. When looking at two objects with single-syllable names, chooses the correct object when it is said with a separation between onset and rime.	SLP: **Each of you is holding a stuffed animal. We have named their body parts. Point to your animal's *t-ail*.** S: Points to the animal's tail.
22. After choosing a picture of a single-syllable word, says the word with a separation between onset and rime.	SLP: **You counted 10 objects on the table. Find the *b-ook*. Then you tell the next student what to find.** S: **Here is the *b-ook*.** S: Tells the next student: **Find the *p-an*.**
Short-Term Goal: Blends phonemes into a word after they are given separately: Sound blending	
23. When looking at two pictures, points to the correct picture when the picture is named with separated sounds.	SLP: **We get to play Bingo today. Put a token on *k-u-p*.** S: Puts a token on the picture of a cup.
24. After hearing a word segmented into separate sounds, says the whole word.	SLP: **Before you take a turn in the game, tell me what word I am trying to say: *b-l-ue*.** S: **Blue**

Objectives	Examples
25. Takes turns with a friend giving words with segmented phonemes and guessing the whole word.	SLP: **Would you like to play the teacher today? You will take turns saying or blending the sounds in sports words: What is this word? *S-o-cc-er.*** S1: **Soccer. What's this word? *T-e-nn-i-s.*** S2: **Tennis. *B-a-se-b-a-ll.*** S3: **Baseball. Then, *f-oo-t-b-a-ll.***
26. After hearing a word that has a consonant blend, segments it into its separate sounds (phonemes).	SLP: **Now let's segment words that have consonant blends. Say the sounds in *spoon.*** S: ***S-p-oo-n***
Short-Term Goal: Adds or deletes a given sound from a word and says the new word or syllable: Sound addition or deletion	
27. Follows instructions to say a word and then says the word again with an added sound to make a new word.	SLP: **Say *oat*. Then say it again, but put /b/ at the beginning.** S: **Oat, boat**
28. Follows instructions to say a word, then says it again with a specified missing sound.	SLP: **Now we will omit a sound. Say *run*. Now say it again, but don't say /r/.** S: **Un**
29. Listens to a word and then says that word with a missing initial or final sound.	SLP: **Listen to this word: *jump*. Now say it again, but don't say the last sound.** S: **Jum**
Short-Term Goal: Adds or substitutes a specified sound in a word and says the new word: Sound substitution	
30. Names a pictured word, then creates a new word by substituting a specific initial sound.	SLP: **Let's make new words out of your spelling words. Name this picture.** S: **Dog** SLP: **Now say it again, but say /f/ instead of /d/.** S: **Fog**
31. After hearing a word, creates a new word by substituting a specific final sound.	SLP: **Before you take a turn at the game, say *game*. Now say it again, but say /t/ instead of /m/.** S: **Gate**
Short-Term Goal: Says the individual sounds in CVC words: Sound segmentation	
32. Repeats after the SLP the phonemes in a one-syllable word.	SLP: **This wild animal is a *bear*. Repeat the sounds in *bear* after me: *b-ea-r*.** S: ***B-ea-r***
33. After hearing a one-syllable word pronounced, says the individual phonemes in the word.	SLP: **Here are some real fruits and vegetables. I want you to point to a fruit. Then say its sounds.** S: Points to a peach and says ***p-ea-ch***.

Reading Accuracy: Grades 1–5

Yearly Goal: *To become an accurate reader by knowing and applying grade-level phonics and word analysis skills in decoding words*

CCSS.ELA-LITERACY.RF.1.3–RF.5.3
CCSS.ELA-LITERACY.RF.2.3.D

Objectives	Examples
1. Shows knowledge of one-to-one letter–sound correspondences by saying the sound for each consonant.	SLP: **Say the consonant sound on each card.** S: **p, b, t, d, k, g, f, v, s, z, j, m, n, l**
2. Produces the long and short sounds for the five major vowels.	SLP: **Turn over a vowel card and say the sound of each short or long vowel sound.** S: **a, e, i, o, u, a-e, e-e, i-e, o-e, u-e**
3. Recognizes and reads words with common grade-level final consonant digraphs.	SLP: **Some of the words in this list have consonant digraphs. Circle the words I say that have consonant digraphs. Then read the words you circled.** S: **Taps, bits, act, digs, fist, crisp, mask, felt**
4. Memorizes and reads common high-frequency sight words, such as *the, of, she, my, is, are, do, does.*	SLP: **Sight words do not follow the rules that most words do. Read the sight words on these cards over and over until you can read them quickly and easily.** S: **Their, wash, many, buy, done, show, own**
5. Decodes regularly spelled one-syllable CV and CVC words in short sentences.	SLP: **Read the words on your list. Each word has a consonant–vowel or consonant–vowel–consonant. Read the words. Then read the sentence.** S: **Go, me, sat, pet, Kip, hop, fun, root. Tom can pet his cat.**
6. Practices the *final -e rule* for long vowel sounds in syllables or pseudowords.	SLP: **Let's practice the *final -e rule*. Read each syllable these tiles make when I change the letter *e* tile and *f* tile.** S: **afe, aff, afe, aff, afe, afe, aff, afe, aff**
7. Applies the *final -e rule* when reading passages and words, such as *lake, site, mole.*	SLP: **Use the *final -e rule* as you read these sentences with your partner.** S: **Mike rode his bike to Jon's home.**
8. Reads common vowel team conventions for long vowel sounds, such as *coat, eat, say.*	SLP: **We will practice the vowel teams *oa, ea, ay.* Read the list of words on the board. Then read the sentence.** S: **Seal, soap, play. "I have a pet seal," Ray said to Jean.**

Objectives	Examples
9. Recognizes the two short words within compound words, and puts them together to form new words, such as *houseboat*, *popcorn*, *pillbox*.	SLP: **Here are cards that have short, single words. (1) Read the short words on the cards. (2) Then put two short words together to make a longer word.** S: **(1) some, fast, day, book, store, break; (2) someday, breakfast, bookstore**
10. Understands that every syllable must have a vowel sound to determine the number of syllables in a printed word.	SLP: **Your work sheet has a list of two- and three-syllable words. Remember that every syllable must have a vowel. Underline each syllable in these words. Then read the words.** S: Underlines and reads *un-der*, *ad-ven-ture*.
11. Decodes two-syllable words.	SLP: **The words on the board have two syllables. Draw a line on each word to show the two syllables. Clap as you say the syllables. Then say the word.** S: (claps while saying each syllable) **af-ter, after; run-ning, running; pass-ing, passing**
12. Applies knowledge of word roots and common prefixes, such as *un*, *mis-*, *im-*, to read words, such as *uncommon*, *mistake*, *import*.	SLP: **Your work sheet has a list of prefixes (*un-*, *re-*, *in-*, *dis-*, *pre-*, *tele-*) and a list of root or base words (*come*, *lock*, *active*, *read*, *write*, *test*, *like*, *phone*). Match a prefix with a root word to make a new word.** S: (matches and reads) **unlock, reread, income, dislike, pretest, telephone**
13. Applies knowledge of word roots and common suffixes, such as *-ing*, *-less*, *-ward*, to read words, such as *walking*, *countless*, *inward*.	SLP: **Here are sets of cards with four root words and four word endings. Read the root words and the endings. See how many words you can make.** S: **The root words are *play*, *work*, *watch*, *teach*. The suffixes are *-ing*, *-er*, *-est*, *-ful*. My words are *teacher*, *watching*, *playful*, *worker*.**
14. Distinguishes long and short vowels when reading regularly spelled one-syllable words.	SLP: **I want you to write some words on your paper. On line 1 write the words with short vowels. On line 2, write the words with long vowels. Now read all of the words.** S: **On line 1, I wrote *tap*, *cod*, *leg*, *rip*, *pup*. On line 2, I wrote *cute*, *tile*, *meet*, *tote*, *gate*.**
15. Takes apart and reads two-syllable words that have two consonants surrounded by two vowels, such as *goblet*, *mitten*, *attic*, *magnet*, *happens*, *tablet*.	SLP: **Break these words between the consonants: *goblin*, *funny*, *mittens*. Then use the words to write a sentence. Read the words and the sentence.** S: ***gob-lin*, *fun-ny*, *mit-tens*. The goblin in the story has funny mittens.**

(continues)

Objectives	Examples
16. Reads grade-appropriate irregularly spelled words (sight words).	SLP: **Read the sight words on your cards. Sort the cards into two stacks: (1) the words you read quickly and (2) the words you need to practice.** S: Stack 1: *fall, want, put, show, what, grow.* Stack 2: *wash, pull, your, know.*
17. Decodes familiar three-syllable words.	SLP: **Break and read these three-syllable words listed on your paper. Then read the sentence.** S: ***Va-ca-tion, vacation; thun-der-ing, thundering.*** **It was thundering last night.**
18. Reads words that contrast the *soft c* (as in *city, circus*) and *hard c* (as in *cow, come*). *Note:* The letter *c* usually has the sound of *s* when it is followed by the vowels *e, i,* or *y*. This sound is called the *soft* sound of *c*.	SLP: **Read this list of words that have either *soft c* or *hard c* sounds.** S: **Calf, cow, city, cook, circle, circus**
19. Reads words that contrast the *soft g* (as in *gym, giant*) and *hard g* (as in *goat, give*). *Note:* The soft sound of the letter *g* makes the *j* sound when it is followed by *e, i,* or *y*.	SLP: **Read this list of words that have *soft g* or *hard g* sounds.** S: **Giant, goose, general, germ, goes, gentle, guess**
20. Increases amount of time spent reading books at an independent reading level (passages in which the words can be read fluently with 95% accuracy) in order to carry over strategies for decoding accuracy.	SLP: **We will begin making a habit of reading every day for fun. At the library, choose books that are easy to read. Don't pick out hard books, and start a log of the time you spend reading for enjoyment. How do you find an easy book?** S: **Open the book and read a paragraph. If there are lots of words I cannot read, I can look for another book.**

Reading Fluency: Grades 1–12

Yearly Goal: *To support reading comprehension by reading aloud fluently (quickly and accurately with good understanding) and with no need to sound out words part by part*

CCSS.ELA-LITERACY.RF.1.4–RF.5.4

Objectives	Examples
Short-Term Goal: Increases speed in quickly recognizing and reading frequently occurring written letter patterns	
1. Quickly recognizes and reads written consonant letter patterns in words, sentences, and brief passages in which the patterns occur frequently. *Note:* Letter patterns: VC, CV, CVC, VCC, CCV, CCVC, CVCC, CCVCC.	SLP: **We will practice reading quickly and accurately. These practice times will help your reading comprehension. This list has words that begin with the consonant blend /pr/. Read the list over and over as quickly and accurately as you can.** S: Quickly reads the list over and over for 1 minute: **pray, press, price, prince, prize, problem.**

Objectives	Examples
2. Quickly recognizes and reads written vowel letter patterns (i.e., two-letter vowel combinations) in words, sentences, and brief passages in which the patterns occur frequently.	SLP: **All of the words in this list have the target vowel digraph *ea*. Read the list of words quickly and accurately over and over until the timer goes off.** S: **Beak, deal, read, sea, neat, leap, teach, easy**
Short-Term Goal: Increases speed in quickly recognizing and reading frequently occurring syllable and word patterns	
3. Quickly recognizes and reads simple and complex syllable patterns in words, sentences, and brief passages in which the patterns occur frequently.	SLP: **I want you to read aloud these two lists of simple CVC words and silent *e* words. Quickly read the two lists for 1 minute. Then read the short paragraph with the same words in it.** S: Quickly reads the words, then the paragraph: **(1) cap, lad, cot, root, leg, pat; (2) face, ate, poke, June, cave.**
4. Quickly recognizes and reads morpheme patterns in words, sentences, and brief passages in which the patterns occur frequently.	SLP: **Look at this list of word beginnings. Quickly read the list many times. Then read the words that contain the same prefixes.** S: Reads over and over: **mega-, meta-, photo-, pano-, tele-, metro.** Then reads over and over: **megaphone, metatarsus, photographer, panorama, telephone, metropolitan.**
5. Quickly recognizes and reads multisyllabic words that contain prefixes and suffixes.	SLP: **Read this list of words aloud.** S: **Lunches, recognize, unhappy, curriculum, assignment, classification**
6. Quickly recognizes and reads sight words.	SLP: **This list contains target sight words you have studied. Read it quickly and accurately: *hold, wash, know, fall, does*. Quickly read the words, then read the short paragraph until the timer goes off.** S: Reads **hold, wash, know, fall, does,** then reads the paragraph.
Short-Term Goal: Increases vocabulary and passage comprehension to improve reading fluency	
7. Selects and previews meanings of key words before reading a passage.	SLP: **Explain the meaning of key words in this passage. Then set the timer and take turns reading the passage with your partner. Don't stop until you hear the timer.**
8. Increases understanding of words with multiple meanings.	SLP: **Tell as many meanings as possible for each of these multiple-meaning words. Then make up a sentence for the word.** S: ***Roll* can mean to move forward by turning over and over. *Roll* can mean a round piece of bread. Sentence: I like to put butter and honey on a roll.**

(continues)

Objectives	Examples
9. Responds accurately to comprehension questions. Then rereads for *repeated oral reading* a passage in which 19 of 20 words (95%) can be read correctly and easily.	SLP: **Read this paragraph about Sojourner Truth. Find out what her name means.** S: **It means traveler-for-truth.** SLP: **You read 95% of the words correctly! You may take your paragraph home to practice for your daily repeated oral reading.**
Short-Term Goal: Increases reading rate in context	
10. Increases speed and accuracy by repeat reading.	SLP: **You have read this story passage with 95% accuracy. I want you to read the passage again and again for 1 minute. Each time, try to read further with fewer errors.** S: Reads for 1 minute, going further each time.
11. Increases speed and accuracy by focusing attention on the printed words or sentence structure.	SLP: **Pay close attention to each word in this sentence. Read the sentence from back to front then front to back. Now read it over and over for 1 minute.** S: Reads sentence back to front then front to back for 1 minute.
12. Increases speed and accuracy by focusing attention on meaning.	SLP: **Read this short newspaper article. Pay close attention to the meaning. When you notice something that doesn't make sense, stop and correct it.** S: **In 1787, there were 13 *skates* . . . there were 13 states.**
13. Increases speed and accuracy by improving attention to syntactic structure and prosody (i.e., intonation, stress, pause, juncture, rhythm, and timing).	SLP: **Listen to me read this paragraph. Now you read it and try to make it sound like I did. Think about where I paused, my intonation, and the rhythm.** S: Imitates the reading.
Short-Term Goal: Increases the natural flow of oral reading through practice and repetition	
14. Increases speed and accuracy by regularly reading the same story to younger students.	SLP: **Choose a book that was your favorite when you were younger. Now go and read it to each of the kindergarten classes.** S: Reads *The Gingerbread Boy*.
15. Increases speed and accuracy by responding to ongoing teacher feedback and guidance regarding oral reading.	SLP: **How would you say the sentence "Close the door, please" to someone? Look at me and say, "Close the door, please." Now read it aloud with the same intonation and pauses.** S: Reads the sentence with conversational expression.

Objectives	Examples
16. Increases speed and accuracy by practicing daily oral reading of short passages that can be read with ease (at the independent reading level with 19 of 20 words correct) at least 15 minutes per day.	SLP: **Take turns with your partner reading aloud this passage from your social studies book.** S: Reads a selected passage with 95% accuracy, practices it daily for several days, and receives a new passage as needed.
17. Develops oral reading automaticity by practicing lyrics to songs.	SLP: **Work with your group to choose a favorite song. Then print out the lyrics. Practice reading the lyrics out loud with your group. Next week, you will present your song reading to the rest of the class.**

Reading Comprehension of Literature: Grades 1–3

Yearly Goal: *To read and understand various literary forms (e.g., sentences, poems, picture books, stories, grade-level texts)*

CCSS.ELA-LITERACY.RL.1.7–RL.3.7
CCSS.ELA-LITERACY.RL.1.1–RL.3.1
CCSS.ELA-LITERACY.RL.1.3–RL.3.3
CCSS.ELA-LITERACY.RL.1.4–RL.3.4
CCSS.ELA-LITERACY.RL.3.9

Objectives	Examples
Short-Term Goal: Determines the key ideas and details	
1. Makes predictions about what the story may be about based on the book cover and illustrations.	SLP: **Look at our new book! Let's look at the cover and some of the pictures. What do you think the story will be about?** S: **I see pictures of an elephant and a tiger. Maybe the book is about jungle animals.**
2. Asks and answers questions to show understanding of a text, using the text as a basis for the answer.	SLP: **Look on this page of our book. Read the sentence that tells what happened to the dog.** S: Points to the answer and reads, **The dog found his bone.**
3. Asks and answers questions about key details in a text.	SLP: **Did you like our new story? Ask the person next to you some questions about the title, the main character, and one thing that happened in our new book.** S: Takes turns asking and answering questions about key details of the book.

(continues)

Objectives	Examples
4. Retells stories, including key details and the central message, lesson, or moral.	SLP: **Let's take turns as we go around the circle retelling the story *The Rainbow Fish*.** S1: **Rainbow Fish has pretty scales.** S2: **He is lonely. He doesn't have any friends.** S3: **He learned to share his sparkly scales.** S4: **He made new friends.**
5. Describes characters, settings, and major events in a story using key details.	SLP: **When you practice your oral book report, remember to tell about the characters in your book, where the story takes place, and what happens in the book.** S: ***The Very Hungry Caterpillar* is about a caterpillar. It takes place near a tree. First it's a tiny seed, then a hungry caterpillar that eats lots of food. He spins a cocoon and turns into a butterfly!**
6. Makes predictions about events and information based on the content of the text.	SLP: **Before we read any more of the story, what do you think will happen next?** S: **If everything turns to gold, Midas won't have anything to eat!**
7. Describes how characters in a story respond to major events and challenges.	SLP: **How do you think Papa Bear sounded when he saw his bedspread wrinkled and some of his porridge eaten? What would he do?** S: **I think he would be mad. He would try to find out who had been in his house, and the next time he left he would be sure to lock the door.**
8. Describes characters in a story, including their traits, motivations, or feelings, and explains how their actions contribute to the sequence of events.	SLP: **Let's talk about Mouse in the story *If You Give a Mouse a Cookie*. What does he want? How does he feel in different times of the story? Does he stick with one thing or do many things?** S: **The mouse in this story was very busy. He wanted a cookie and a glass of milk but then began many other activities. He was happy, sleepy, and distracted.**
Short-Term Goal: Craft and structure: Interprets words and phrases and figurative language	
9. Determines the meanings of words and characters' behaviors that suggest feelings.	SLP: **When reading, it helps to know about the characters' feelings. Let's talk about some actions or words that help us decide how the characters feel. Tell me how you would know that a character was tired. We will write words on the left and behaviors on the right.** S: **Words: *exhausted*, *weary*, and *fatigued*. Actions: *walking slowly*, *nodding the head*, *closing eyes*, and *lying down*.**

Objectives	Examples
10. Identifies who is telling the story at different points in the story.	SLP: **David, you read the part of the dragon. Allison, you read the part of the princess.** S: Students read their parts in voices to match the speakers.
11. Describes how words and phrases, such as repeated lines, lend meaning and rhythm in a story.	SLP: **Let's read this part aloud together: "I think I can, I think I can." What does that repeated phrase remind you of in the story?** S: **It makes me think of the wheels of the train turning and making it up the hill.**
12. Distinguishes literal from nonliteral language, as in "shake a leg."	SLP: **We sometimes use phrases that don't mean exactly what we say. If I look out the window and say, "It's raining cats and dogs," what do I mean?** S: **You mean it's raining very hard.**
Short-Term Goal: Integration of knowledge and ideas: Illustrations, comparing stories	
13. Uses information gained from illustrations and words in print to add meaning to the story.	SLP: **Let's look at the pictures and print on this page. What do they tell us about the story?** S: **The pictures tell us that it is winter. The large print means to read it with a loud voice, and the tiny print is for a soft voice.**
14. Compares and contrasts themes, settings, and characters in different books written by the same author. *Note:* Refer to the compare-and-contrast visual organizer in Appendix C.	SLP: **Have a reporter from your group tell us about how our two different Ellie books are alike and different.** S: **They are alike because Ellie met new people and had a good time. They are different because Ellie went to a farm and met the farmer and cows in the first book. In the second book, she visited kindergarten, met kids, and played with them on the playground.**

Reading Comprehension of Literature: Grades 4–8

Yearly Goal: *To read and understand various literary forms (fairy tales, stories, myths, poems, picture books, fantasies, fictional stories, chapter books, science fiction, tall tales, mysteries, novels, and plays)*

CCSS.ELA-LITERACY.RL.4.2–RL.8.2
CCSS.ELA-LITERACY.RL.4.1
CCSS.ELA-LITERACY.RL.4.7–RL.6.7
CCSS.ELA-LITERACY.RL.5.3 and RL.6.3

Note: See Appendix C for the story map visual organizer.

Objectives	Examples
Short-Term Goal: Before beginning to read, makes a connection with the story and the purpose for reading it	
1. Predicts what a story will be about by examining the book's title, author, cover, illustrations, and chapter titles.	SLP: **Look carefully at the title, pictures, and book cover in *The Keeping Quilt*. What do you think the story might be about?** S: **It might be about a family's quilt.**
2. Before reading a classroom text, explains whether the reason for reading is for pleasure or to find factual information.	SLP: **Think about why we will read this book. Is it for pleasure or to find out factual information?** S: **The pictures and cover show us it's a book to read for pleasure.**
3. Predicts what could happen to the main character or how a mystery or problem could be solved by scanning the text and pictures.	SLP: **You decided that *A Wrinkle in Time* will be about traveling through time. List problems that characters might confront.** S: (writes) Where to get food. How to survive outer space. How to stay in touch with people on Earth.
4. Determines a story theme or central idea and relates the theme to previous knowledge about the theme or previously read books or stories.	SLP: **The theme of our new story is freedom. Think of other stories we have with a *freedom* theme.** S: ***Johnny Tremain* was a book about paying the price to fight for freedom.**
5. Locates potentially difficult or unfamiliar words by scanning the text.	SLP: **Scan the first chapter to find words you don't yet know. I'll list them on the board.** S: **I found the words *prodigious* and *placid*.**
6. Establishes personal reason or purpose for reading a story or book.	SLP: **Look through the new library book you chose. Write down your own reason for choosing it.** S: (writes) I want to read *My Side of the Mountain* to find out how Sam, a boy my age, could survive winter all alone in the Catskill Mountains.

Objectives	Examples
Short-Term Goal: Becomes actively involved in the story right from the beginning in order to get the general gist of the story	
7. Establishes from the beginning the story's location, time period, and names of characters.	SLP: **Scan your new book, *The Upstairs Room*, and jot down names of characters, places, dates, and seasons in the first three chapters.** S: (writes) fall, 1938, Germany, Sini, Rachel, the Ganses
8. Establishes the *wh-* questions (who, what, where, when, and why) in a story from the beginning and cites the information in the text.	SLP: **Underline sentences on your page that answer this question: Why do you think the narrator gave up a brilliant career in painting?** S: Underlines the text.
9. From time to time, stops to summarize the plot to recount the sequence of events.	SLP: **Before we begin episode 3 in *Rainbow Crow*, tell what happened in episode 2.** S: **The animals came together to decide which one would travel to the Great Sky.**
10. From time to time, stops to tell the main idea in a paragraph.	SLP: **Tell us what this paragraph is mostly about.** S: **James names his new puppy Major.**
11. Uses imagery or visualization to understand interactions of time, settings, and characters in a story.	SLP: **Imagine the setting for the millhouse that Sam Gribley described in *On the Far Side of the Mountain*. Draw a map and label the mountain, stream, and millhouse.** S: Creates and labels a map.
12. Describes the overall structure of a story, including beginning, middle, and ending episodes, or significant events.	SLP: **Draw a time line of the story we just read. Write the words *beginning, middle,* and *end* on the time line. Also write words to indicate important things that happened in the story, showing on the time line when they occurred.** S: (writes on time line) (1) Sam's cat is lost. (2) A fireman rescues his cat. (3) His cat is home again.
Short-Term Goal: Goes beyond given information in the text to analyze text and discover deeper meanings	
13. Analyzes characters, settings, dates, problems, solutions, and concluding events. *Note:* See Appendix C for the story map visual organizer.	SLP: **Work with your partner to complete a story map. On the map, enter the characters' names, setting, dates, problems, solutions, and story outcome.** S: Enters information.
14. Compares and contrasts characters, settings, and events.	SLP: **Let's compare two important characters in Jess's world, Leslie and Miss Edwards. They were very different characters but were alike in some ways. Tell some ways they were alike.** S: **Both inspired him to do his best. Each one had a good sense of humor. Both admired him.**

(continues)

Objectives	Examples
15. Compares and contrasts a written story to the same story presented in a movie or play.	SLP: **You've read the book and seen the movie *Bridge to Terabithia*. Compare your experiences.** S: **In the movie, I liked seeing the real bridge and the river, but I enjoyed the book more. It showed better how Jess could survive his friend's death. Leslie was his bridge to discover his strength.**
16. Explains how characters in a story change as they respond to challenges.	SLP: **In our book, *A Wrinkle in Time*, what events caused Charles Wallace to change after he tried to find out about the man with red eyes?** S: **Charles Wallace felt his sister Meg's genuine love for him. Meg's love broke the evil man's control over him.**
17. Identifies with characters in the story and imagines acting in ways similar to those of the characters.	SLP: **In our short story, Emily agreed to stand in to sing a solo for her friend Lea, who got sick. Despite Emily's fears, she practiced hard and sang well. Suppose you were afraid to do something. How would you overcome your fears?** S: **I would practice hard. I would imagine myself doing well and seeing others cheering for me.**
18. Tells how characters responded and felt at different times in the story and supports the ideas with reasons.	SLP: **Think about how Emily's friend Lea may have felt at different times in the story. Tell three ways she felt, and give the reasons.** S: **Lea felt proud when she won the solo part, disappointed when she got sick, and relieved that Emily offered to stand in for her.**
19. Draws conclusions after combining information from different parts of the story.	SLP: **In our story, little Matt colored all over his cousin Sam's math homework. When Sam saw it he yelled, "You're ruining my math paper! Get out of here, you little creep!" Matt started to cry. Why?** S: **Matt felt terrified when he heard Sam yelling and saw Sam shaking his fist at him.**
20. Organizes themes or central ideas in the story according to changes in time periods in the story.	SLP: **Leslie's accident was a pivotal point in the book. How did Leslie's accident affect Jess? Make two columns to list the changes.** S: Left column: before the accident—courageous, brave, hopeful Right column: after the accident—depressed, despondent, reclusive
21. Organizes themes and central ideas in the story according to changes in characters' feelings or relationships.	SLP: **How do you think Jess will be a different adult as a result of knowing Leslie?** S: **Jess often felt angry, fearful, and frustrated. Leslie's friendship gave him courage. As an adult he will courageously follow his dreams and accept challenges.**

Objectives	Examples
Short-Term Goal: Synthesizes information gained from the text to make applications, inferences, and predictions and develop new ideas	
22. Applies what has been learned from the text to his or her own life.	SLP: **In *Bridge to Terabithia*, Leslie was a bridge for Jess. Suppose you were a bridge for someone. Tell about it.** S: **I would offer encouragement by listening and cheering them on when they felt afraid or discouraged.**
23. Makes inferences based on given information and previously gained information.	SLP: **Explain how the music teacher, Mr. Roman, felt at different times in the story. What actions showed his feelings?** S: **He felt angry when the stage risers were missing. He folded his arms across his chest and his face was red. He felt relieved after Lisa explained the problem. A big smile spread across his face, and he sighed with relief.**
24. Makes predictions about a future event based on the story.	SLP: **Predict what Jess will do to be a bridge for his younger sister, May Belle, in the future.** S: **Jess will help May Belle believe in herself just as Leslie encouraged him.**
25. Creates something new based on the story.	SLP: **Draw a picture, write a poem, or plan a role play to capture the central messages of the story we just read.** S: **I will write a poem about friendship.**
26. Uses fantasy to change a story part or create a new ending.	SLP: **Suppose Leslie had not moved to Jess's town that summer. How would the story be different?** S: **Jess might not have discovered how courageous he could be.**

Reading Comprehension of Informational Text: Grades 4–8

Yearly Goal: *To read, understand, and gain information from various informational texts—signs, captions, warning labels, written directions and procedures, textbooks, biographies, letters, magazine articles, websites, dictionaries, reference books*

CCSS.ELA-LITERACY.RH.6–8.8
CCSS.ELA-LITERACY.CCRA.R.5
CCSS.ELA-LITERACY.RI.4.7–RI.7.7
CCSS.ELA-LITERACY.RI.4.4–RI.8
CCSS.ELA-LITERACY.RI.8.4
CCSS.ELA-LITERACY.RI.4.2–RI.8.2
CCSS.ELA-LITERACY.RI.6.6–RI.8.6

Objectives	Examples
1. Differentiates fact from opinion accurately and independently.	SLP: **Today we will talk about differences between facts and opinions in what we read. A fact is something that can be proven: The sun is hot. An opinion tells how someone feels or thinks: It's a great day! On this work sheet, underline words that signal information that is likely to be an opinion as opposed to a fact.** S: (underlines) *should, like, feel, best, worst, great*
2. Knows the purpose for reading the directions before beginning to read an assignment.	SLP: **Today you will begin your science project. Before you read for information, read this page of directions for your project. Then read the directions again and underline the words that tell how to complete the assignment. Why is it important to read directions carefully before you start to work?** S: **You make mistakes and waste time if you don't read the directions first.** Reads the directions then underlines the words.
3. Understands the organizational structures of various types of text.	SLP: **Tell how the organization of your social studies book, *Our Country*, is different from that of your biography of Abraham Lincoln.** S: **My social studies book has 26 chapters about U.S. geography and history. There are many colorful maps, charts, graphs, and time lines. My Abraham Lincoln biography is mostly printed text with a black-and-white drawing of Lincoln at the beginning of each of the 10 chapters. The whole book is about Lincoln's life.**

Objectives	Examples
4. Anticipates where information in a classroom text can be found because of an understanding of how the text is organized.	SLP: **In your classroom, you are preparing to write a report about your home state. What do you know about classroom textbooks that will help you locate information about your state?** S: **I know to look in the index to find which pages tell about my state. Scanning the table of contents and the headings in the chapters will guide me to information. There are pictures and charts that will also give me information.**
5. Interprets information presented visually or orally and quantitatively in charts, graphs, diagrams, time lines, and so on.	SLP: **Let's find out what we can learn about Indians from the colorful map on page 14 in your textbook. We easily see which Native American Indian tribes that lived east of the Mississippi River were moved to present-day Oklahoma. Find the tribe that moved to Indian Territory from Tennessee.** S: **Cherokee**
6. Determines the meaning of words and phrases as they are used in a text.	SLP: **Did you enjoy reading about the life of Helen Keller? Look at the sentence "Helen dedicated her life to helping people who could not see or hear." From what you know about Helen, what do you think the word *dedicated* means? If you don't know the word, how could you find out its meaning?** S: **I could look in a dictionary or on the Internet, but I think *dedicated* means that she gave up her life to help others who, like her, couldn't see or hear. She learned to read with her fingers, to write, and even to speak.**
7. Identifies central or main ideas of a text and supporting details accurately and independently.	SLP: **Read the first paragraph in this copy of a page from your science book. Underline the main idea, and then look for supporting ideas.** S: (underlines) (1) easy to recognize swallowtail butterflies, (2) wings with patterns, (3) blue and red spots
8. Determines an author's points of view and purpose in a text.	SLP: **You said that you have a new puppy to train, and I see that you borrowed the library book *No Bad Dogs*. How did the author's point of view help you choose that particular dog-training book?** S: **Yes, I do have a new puppy. The author is a dog trainer herself, and the book has pictures of her training her dogs. The pictures and her writing tell me that she loves and respects dogs. I want to learn from that point of view.**

Unit 8

Literacy: Writing

- Writing Mechanics: Grades K–7
- Writing With Appropriate Form and Style: Grades 3–6
- Writing to Communicate: Grades 1–8
- Writing Process: Grades 1–8

Literacy includes all aspects of language: listening, speaking, reading, and writing. Both spoken and written language share four similarities: (a) At least two people are needed for communication to occur. Speakers need listeners, and writers need readers. (b) A reason is needed to communicate (pragmatics). (c) Both communicate meaning (semantics). (d) A structure is required, phonetic or graphic, to carry the message (syntax and morphology). All of these components are part of literacy.

For many students with language disorders, writing their thoughts is the most difficult aspect of language development. This difficulty is due in part to the higher cognitive demands of writing (Richard, 2001). It is also related to the demands of writing that differ from the demands of speaking. First, in written language, the reader is not present to interact with the writer. Second, written language is more formal, and writers and readers must depend only on words to convey meaning rather than on immediate context or nonverbal cues. Written language also emphasizes different types of sentence and text-level complexity.

Students who become competent writers master a cognitive-linguistic process and produce a written product (American Speech-Language-Hearing Association, 2001). Competency is difficult. Gleason and Ratner (2013) concluded, "Although many students in grades four through twelve can master the basics of writing, far fewer—only about 25 percent—can write proficiently" (p. 353). To master the writing process, students must plan and prewrite, write a first draft, and then revise and rewrite. Finally, they publish a piece of writing, the written product. Publication may be as simple as sharing the paper with a friend or teacher or as advanced as having it published in a student magazine. A written product may be examined and described in several ways. At the word level are word choice and spelling. At the sentence level are grammar, complexity, and style. At the text level are structure and cohesive devices. The written product can also be described according to writing conventions (capitalization, punctuation, paragraphing), its purpose (to entertain or inform), and its effectiveness (influence on its readers).

Writing pulls together ideas, images, disorganized information, and bits and pieces of experiences. Students with language disorders find this synthesis of information difficult (Wiig & Wilson, 1994). In addition, they often struggle with handwriting and spatial arrangement of their writing on a page. They need support in all aspects of the writing process and production of a written product. Speech–language pathologists (SLPs) can provide special help at the prewriting stage by helping students externalize their thoughts. The SLP can ask questions such as these to help with this process: Who will read this paper? What do the readers know? What do the readers need to know? Why are you writing? (Graham & Harris, 1999). Talking about their writing before beginning to write helps students step away from their abbreviated, inner speech to gain a more objective view of writing. SLPs can offer assistance by providing structure while students organize information.

Concept maps as visual organizers have proven especially helpful to organization (see the visual organizers in Appendix C). SLPs can also be supportive to students who need to master writing by being aware of grade-level requirements for spelling, capitalization, punctuation, and paragraph writing. They need to be aware of the writing purposes emphasized at the student's grade level, such as narrative, expository, and persuasive purposes (see Appendix E, "Purposes for Writing," for descriptions of each).

Students with dyslexia and language disorders often struggle with dysgraphia and have special problems with handwriting. *Dysgraphia* is defined as "a writing pattern characterized by substantial effort which interferes with a student's ability to convert ideas into a written format" (Richards, 1999, p. 72). Because of weak motor memory, students with dysgraphia must think about the formation of letters each time they write them. For these students, mastering the sequence of the muscle motor movements needed in writing letters or numbers is not automatic. For students with dysgraphia, computers are a gift. Keyboarding is frequently recommended to help them compensate (Shaywitz, 2003). Students with dysgraphia also benefit when given a writing structure for constructing sentences and writing paragraphs. (Examples of these writing structures are provided in Appendix F, "Writing Frames.")

Description of Contents

Writing Mechanics: Grades K–7. This section provides objectives for some of the basic writing skills, beginning with writing letters of the alphabet and one's own name. The purpose of these objectives is to help develop skills that are important to producing a readable piece for a reader; those skills include age-appropriate handwriting, spelling, and basic punctuation skills.

Writing With Appropriate Form and Style: Grades 3–6. The purpose of these literacy objectives is to help students use age-appropriate grammar and syntax, use clear pronoun referents, and produce a cohesive, logical piece by using transitional and connective words.

Writing to Communicate: Grades 1–8. The objectives are designed to help students consider their reasons for writing and to consider the audience that will read it. Objectives begin with simple reasons to write, such as writing lists and writing notes to friends or family. They extend to objectives for keeping a journal, writing essay test responses, expressing original ideas and humor, and composing research papers and critical analysis essays.

Writing Process: Grades 1–8. This section provides objectives that help students develop a perspective of themselves as writers. Objectives are designed for students at any grade level to plan what they will write, compose a draft, proof their written work, revise and edit it, and, finally, put it into a finished product. These objectives focus on helping students view their writing as a process that will involve planning and making several revisions before it will be ready to share for publication.

The appendixes contain the following materials that may be helpful when planning intervention using the objectives in this unit:

- Appendix B: Conjunctions, transition words, homonyms
- Appendix C: Visual organizers
- Appendix E: Purposes for writing (types)
- Appendix F: Writing frames

Writing Mechanics: Grades K–7

Yearly Goal: *To develop use of age-appropriate legibility, spelling, punctuation, capitalization, neatness, and compensatory methods (e.g., computer, spell-check)*

CCSS.ELA-LITERACY.L.K.1.A and L.1.1.A
CCSS.ELA-LITERACY.L.K.2, L.2.2, L.4.2–L.7
CCSS.ELA-LITERACY.L.K.2.A, L.2.2.A, L.4.2.A
CCSS.ELA-LITERACY.L.K.2.B, L.4.2.B, L.5.2.A–L.5.2.D
CCSS.ELA-LITERACY.L.K.2.D, L.1.2.E, L.2.2.E, L.3.2.G, L.4.2.D, L.5.2.E, L.6.2.B

Objectives	Examples
1. Writes own name.	SLP: **Write your name on your notebooks and classroom papers.** (For students unable to write their names, write the name lightly in dashed lines and have them trace the names.) S: Writes own name to label belongings in the classroom.
2. Writes all letters of the alphabet.	SLP: **On this page, write each letter of the alphabet.** S: Writes each letter of the alphabet.
3. Uses legible handwriting or chooses an appropriate font to enhance the written work.	SLP: **It is important that the writing on your report is neat and easy to read. Let's look at it and see if it can be more legible.** S: Reviews the report with the SLP and writes it again neatly.
4. Uses correct spelling at ability level.	SLP: **How can you be sure that you are spelling the words in your paragraph correctly?** S: **If I am not sure of the spelling of a word, I can look it up in the dictionary or my social studies book or type it into the computer for spell-check.**
5. Uses capitalization and end-of-sentence punctuation rules correctly.	SLP: **Let's review some important points to remember when writing sentences. (1) What kind of letter always starts a sentence? (2) What punctuation goes at the end of (a) a statement, (b) a question, (c) an exciting sentence?** S: **(1) capital letter, (2) (a) period, (b) question mark, (c) exclamation point.** SLP: **Now look at this paragraph and correct the punctuation errors.**

(continues)

Objectives	Examples
6. Capitalizes names, holidays, product names, and geographic names.	SLP: **Look at these four columns. Write some words under each column, starting each with a capital letter: (1) proper names, (2) holidays, (3) product names, (4) geographic names.** S: (writes) (1) Thomas, Mr. Lanza; (2) Christmas, New Year's Day; (3) Crayola, Kleenex; (4) Texas, Mississippi River
7. Selects correct punctuation for the message content.	SLP: **As a group, let's write a short play to present to the rest of the class. When writing it, remember to correctly use quotation marks, commas, apostrophes, and end-of-sentence punctuation.** S: Writes short play with group, paying special attention to correct punctuation.
8. Uses commas to separate items in a series, to separate an introductory element from the rest of the sentence, and to set off the words yes and no.	SLP: **Place commas correctly in the following: (1) My favorite colors are blue green purple and red. (2) At the movies I like to eat popcorn. (3) Yes I love to read.** S: (writes) (1) My favorite colors are blue, green, purple, and red. (2) At the movies, I like to eat popcorn. (3) Yes, I love to read.
9. Uses underlining, quotation marks, or italics to indicate titles of works.	SLP: **The title of this book is *The Cat and The Hat*. Show me the way you could handwrite it to show that it is a title, and how you would type it when using a computer.** S: (writes) The Cat and the Hat, (types) *The Cat and the Hat*
10. Consults a dictionary or computer spell-checker for proofing.	SLP: **Before you turn in your report, be sure to check it for correct spelling.** S: Uses dictionary or computer spell-checker.

Writing With Appropriate Form and Style: Grades 3–6

Yearly Goal: *To write age-appropriate documents with clarity and organization (form) using age-appropriate linguistic rules for forming words, using pronouns, and forming simple and complex sentence patterns (style)*

CCSS.ELA-LITERACY.L.3.3.A
CCSS.ELA-LITERACY.L.4.1.F, L.5.3.A
CCSS.ELA-LITERACY.L.3.2.D
CCSS.ELA-LITERACY.L.3.1.D, L.5.1.C, L.5.1.D
CCSS.ELA-LITERACY.L.5.1, L.5.3, and L.6.3
CCSS.ELA-LITERACY.L.5.1.E
CCSS.ELA-LITERACY.L.4.1.A and L.6.1.D
CCSS.ELA-LITERACY.L.3.1.F
CCSS.ELA-LITERACY.W.3.6
CCSS.ELA-LITERACY.L.6.3.B
CCSS.ELA-LITERACY.W.4.3.C and W.5.3

Objectives	Examples
1. Writes with age-appropriate vocabulary and avoids repeating words or using overworked words (e.g., *very*, *nice*, *cute*, *good*, *bad*, *gonna*).	SLP: **Write a paragraph replacing overworked words with more dynamic adjectives, nouns, and verbs. Replace *I felt happy*.** S: (writes) When my little lost puppy ran to me, I scooped him up and held him close. It thrilled me when he licked my cheek with his warm little tongue!
2. When writing complete sentences, recognizes and corrects inappropriate fragments and run-on sentences.	SLP: **Look at this report from the school talent show. Cross out the sentence fragment, and then write the correct sentence on your work sheet.** S: (writes) Ethan played the piano in the school talent show.
3. When writing, shows distinctions between noun plurals and possessives.	SLP: **Write a sentence about the science lesson that shows distinctions between possessive *s* and plural *s*.** S: (writes) Comparing the sizes of elephants' ears is one way to distinguish African from Asian elephants.
4. When writing, uses regular and irregular verbs appropriately.	SLP: **Correct the sentence on the board to show the correct verb tense: Many soldiers is marching toward the fort.** S: (writes) Many soldiers are marching toward the fort.
5. Writes verb tense correctly to show various times, sequences, states, and conditions.	SLP: **Correct the verb tense errors in the sentence on your work sheet: I went into the hall, and there I see a tall man.** S: (writes) I went into the hall, and there I saw a tall man.

(continues)

Objectives	Examples
6. Uses the correlative conjunctions *neither/nor* and *either/or* correctly when writing.	SLP: **Write a sentence about what you will do after school. Include *neither/nor* and *either/or* in your report.** S: (writes) I will neither walk to school nor ride. I will skate! I will eat either an apple or a banana.
7. When writing, recognizes and corrects inappropriate shifts in verb tense.	SLP: **On your work sheet, correct the incorrect shifts in verb tense in this sentence: I came into the kitchen, and I see a plate of cookies.** S: (writes) I came into the kitchen, and I saw a plate of cookies.
8. Uses pronouns correctly in sentences when writing.	SLP: **Include pronouns when you write a summary of Becca's report on the U.S. Senate.** S: (writes) U.S. citizens of every state elect two senators to represent their state in the U.S. Senate.
9. When writing, corrects errors in the use of pronouns and antecedents.	SLP: **Change the unclear pronouns in this sentence to match their antecedents: Benjamin's brother was married when he was six years old.** S: (writes) Benjamin's brother was married when Benjamin was six years old.
10. Writes questions using the relative pronouns *who, when, what, which, whose.*	SLP: **Use some relative pronouns when writing a *wh-* question for an interview with Benjamin Franklin.** S: (writes) Which of your famous sayings is your favorite, Mr. Franklin?
11. Uses a variety of sentence patterns when writing (e.g., declarative, interrogative, imperative, exclamatory).	SLP: **List the types of sentence patterns you used in your written report.** S: (writes) imperative, declarative, interrogative
12. When writing, stays mindful of reader interest by using appropriate transitional and connective words to link ideas and make transitions (e.g., *then, first, next, after, before, because, since, finally, otherwise*).	SLP: **Write your final paragraph. Use connective and transitional words.** S: (writes) Finally, I am sure it is fortunate that we learn how to talk as children. Otherwise, we might be too discouraged by the difficulties to persevere!
13. Writes with appropriate form to produce a clear and organized document that furthers the quality and purpose of the content, whether written by hand or on a computer.	SLP: **Write a paragraph to describe your plans for writing and publishing your book report.** S: (writes) I will type my book report on the computer. On page 1, I will enter the book title and author. A colorful picture from the Internet will go at the bottom of that page. Finally, I'll enter my summary and conclusion.

Writing to Communicate: Grades 1–8

Yearly Goal: *To apply age-appropriate pragmatic rules to written communication for a variety of readers as indicated by word choices, elaboration, perspective-taking, social register, and creativity*

CCSS.ELA-LITERACY.W.3.3–W.8.3
CCSS.ELA-LITERACY.W.3.10–W.6.10 and W.8.10
CCSS.ELA-LITERACY.W.4.4 and W. 5.4
CCSS.ELA-LITERACY.W.7.2.D and W.8.2.D
CCSS.ELA-LITERACY.W.6.1.D–W.8.1.D

Objectives	Examples
Short-Term Goal: Writes to accomplish a variety of communicative purposes	
1. Uses written language to make requests or respond to requests of others (e.g., lists, letters, notes).	SLP: **Write a letter to your partner requesting something like coming to your party or helping you to organize a fund-raising project. Then, trade letters and write your response. Remember to be polite and specific in both the request and the response.** S: Writes a request letter and a response letter.
2. Completes forms (e.g., questionnaires, club reports, employment applications).	SLP: **Many times, you have to fill out a form for things like a survey or a job application. As you fill out this questionnaire, tell me some things you need to remember.** S: (fills out questionnaire) **I need to write neatly, be honest in my answers, complete all of the questions, and answer the questions in a clear and precise manner.**
3. Writes notes or letters or responds to others' notes and letters for keeping in touch with friends.	SLP: **I want you to write a letter to your pen pal. What are some things you could include that will help you and your pen pal become friends?** S: (writes letter to pen pal) **I could tell her my name and something about my family and things I like to do. I could also ask her some questions to find out more about her.**
4. Writes telephone messages.	SLP: **Pretend you're helping in the school office and receive an important telephone call. Write down the message and deliver it to the proper person. What are some things you need to include?** S: (takes a phone message) **My message needs to have the person's name, a callback phone number, and a brief message. I need to write neatly.**

(continues)

Objectives	Examples
5. Writes directions for making something.	SLP: **Write down the directions for making your craft. Give them to a friend and see if he can follow them. Tell me some things to remember to write in your directions.** S: (writes directions to a craft) **I need to include a list of the materials and number each clearly written step. I should try to follow the directions myself to be sure they are correct.**
6. Writes directions to locations.	SLP: **Look at this map of the city. Write down directions telling how to get from the school on Vista Lane to the public library. Then ask two friends to read your directions and see if they can follow them.** S: (writes) Go out the school front door and turn right on Vista Lane. Go two blocks and turn right on Ramirez Street. Go one block. The library is on the corner of Ramirez and Summer Street.
7. Keeps a journal.	SLP: **Your assignment for the next 3 weeks is to write in a journal for the first 10 minutes of this period. What are some things you could write?** S: Journals for 10 minutes each day in class. **I could write about how my day has gone so far, what I hope to do after school, what my friends and I like to do, or how I'm feeling that day.**
8. Writes a summary.	SLP: **Write a brief summary of the play we just watched. Then, explain your plan for writing it.** S: (writes a brief summary) **I imagined that my readers knew nothing about the play. I gave the title and each major point without explaining details or giving my opinions. I wrote my summary in third person, present tense, as in "Mary writes a letter; then she leaves."**
9. Writes poems, plays, narratives, or expository works for classroom or personal pleasure.	SLP: **Extend what you have been learning in class by writing a poem or story at home. Let's brainstorm some ideas for your poem or story.** S: **I could write a story about my first day at summer camp or how I celebrated my last birthday. I could write a poem comparing two delicious ice cream flavors or about choosing my first pet.**
10. Expresses in writing original ideas, humor, and creativity.	SLP: **Today we are going to work on creative writing. Use your own thoughts and words to write a story that a young child might enjoy. When you are finished, we will choose some of the stories to be read to the kindergarten class.** S: Writes a story about his new puppy.

Objectives	Examples
11. Writes to analyze and interpret a piece of literature in essay form (e.g., Consider this paragraph from *The Adventures of Tom Sawyer* by Mark Twain: "I never seen anybody but lied, one time or another, without it was Aunty Polly—Tom's Aunt Polly, she is—and Mary, and the Widow Douglas, is all told about in that book—which is mostly a true book, with some stretchers, as I said before").	SLP: **Write a section of an essay in which you explain how Mark Twain used voice to help us see the character Huck Finn.** S: (writes) In this paragraph, Mark Twain broke rules left and right to help us experience the character Huckleberry Finn. Notice his terrible grammar. See the way he interrupts himself and repeats himself. He puts us right in the room with Huck Finn.
Short-Term Goal: Provides information by writing answers to test questions	
12. Writes short answers to questions about a section of text.	SLP: **Sometimes a teacher instructs you to write short words or phrases on tests. How will you know when he wants complete sentences or words or phrases? Write your answer.** S: (writes) I will listen carefully to his instructions and read any written instructions. If I still don't know, I will ask a question politely.
13. Restates the question to answer questions about a section of text.	SLP: **Think about the book we just read, *A Wrinkle in Time*. Write a complete sentence that restates the question "Where did Charles Wallace meet the unicorn?"** S: (writes) Charles Wallace met the unicorn near the star-watching rock.
14. Answers essay questions using a paragraph that includes a topic sentence and an appropriate amount of supporting details on the topic.	SLP: **I want you to write a paragraph about this chapter in the book *April Morning*. First, write your topic sentence.** S: (writes) In this chapter, there are two stories going on at the same time, to show the reader where Adam could be instead of where he actually was.
Short-Term Goal: Considers the audience that will read the writing	
15. Recognizes inadequacy based on the audience perspective and adds extra information to make the message complete enough for the intended audience.	SLP: **Think about your reader when you are writing. For example, when you take a test, always check your answers and think about your teacher's perspective. Write down questions you could ask yourself to be sure he will be able to understand your answers.** S: (writes) I will ask myself these questions: Was I specific? Did I give enough information for my teacher to understand my ideas?

(continues)

Objectives	Examples
16. Takes into account the perspective of the audience and the purpose of writing.	SLP: **Write two descriptions of a class play for students who did not see the play, one for a classmate and one for a younger student. Then, tell me how you will find out if your descriptions suited each student's perspective.** S: (writes two descriptions) **When I read my descriptions to the older student and the younger student, I will watch their facial expressions. If they seem bored or confused, I will edit my descriptions.**
17. Writes with appropriate social register and familiarity for the purpose of distinguishing jargon, slang, and informal and formal language.	SLP: **Write an e-mail to a friend about homework and an e-mail to a teacher to request information. Write a paragraph to describe how the two e-mails are different.** S: (writes an e-mail to a friend and then to a teacher) **In my e-mail to my friend, I used casual language and some slang. In my letter to a teacher, I used courteous but formal language.**

Writing Process: Grades 1–8

Yearly Goal: *To apply age-appropriate means to plan, organize, compose, proof, edit, and publish written work in various styles depending on the subject matter, audience, occasion, shared experience, and purpose for writing*

CCSS.ELA-LITERACY.W.K.8–W.4.8
CCSS.ELA-LITERACY.W.3.1.A–W.5.1.A
CCSS.ELA-LITERACY.W.3.3–W.5.3, W.3.3.C–W.5.3.C
CCSS.ELA-LITERACY.W.4.2.D and W. 5.2.D, W.4.3.D and W.5.3.D
CCSS.ELA-LITERACY.W.3.1–W.5.1
CCSS.ELA-LITERACY.W.3.2.B–W.5.2.B
CCSS.ELA-LITERACY.W.3.1.D–W.5.1.D, W.4.2.E and W.5.2.E, W. 3.3.D, W.3.3.E–W.5.3.E
CCSS.ELA-LITERACY.W.4.2.C and W.5.2.C
CCSS.ELA-LITERACY.W.4.3.C and W.5.3.C
CCSS.ELA-LITERACY.W.3.2–W.5.2
CCSS.ELA-LITERACY.W.K.5–W.5.5
CCSS.ELA-LITERACY.W.K.6–W.8.6
CCSS.ELA-LITERACY.W.3.4–W.5.4

Note: See the visual organizers in Appendix C for concept maps to help in planning these objectives.

Objectives	Examples
Short-Term Goal: Develops prewriting skills to plan and prepare for writing	
1. Identifies the purpose of the proposed writing and the audience to be addressed (narrative, descriptive, persuasive, expository).	SLP: **To write a good research report, you need to decide on the purpose of your report. What are some questions you could ask before you start to write about this person?** S: **What is the purpose of my report? Tell a story? Describe the person? Persuade the reader to do something after reading the report? Give information about this person's life?**
2. Selects a writing voice (decides how to *say it*).	SLP: **Before you write a report about a personal experience, you need to decide how to say it. This is called a writing voice. List some ways you could tell your story.** S: **My writing voice could be friendly, humorous, formal, casual, satirical, descriptive, or informative.**
3. Generates and develops ideas or experiences for writing.	SLP: **Let's think of ways you can find evidence when writing a letter to support your opinion.** S: **I could look at pictures, brainstorm, read books, do research, make lists, make visual organizers, interview people, or search reliable Web sites.**

(continues)

Objectives	Examples
4. Creates visual organizers (e.g., story maps, characterization maps, episode maps, simple causal maps, compare and contrast maps, webs, diagrams, drawings) or outlines to organize information concretely and visually.	SLP: **Here is an idea for helping you create a main character for a narrative. Imagine this person in your mind and make a visual organizer like the one on the board to develop his traits. Draw a box in the center of your page. Write your main character's name in it. Draw eight boxes surrounding the name. Write an adjective that describes him in each box.** S: Draws and fills in a characterization map. **My character is Josh. I wrote these adjectives to describe him. He is *impulsive, active, fluent, smart-mouthed, sometimes defiant, respectful, intelligent, a good sport.***
5. Categorizes and organizes the ideas that were gathered.	SLP: **Write a narrative to continue the story we just read in class. Think about the things you want to put in your narrative, and then plan your story in sequence of what you think could happen from beginning, to middle, to end.** S: Writes ideas in three columns labeled *beginning*, *middle*, and *end*.
6. Develops a logical order for presenting the ideas by sequencing and outlining.	SLP: **I want you to write a description of your classmate. After you interview a partner, outline the information you gained and organize it in an outline or put it in the form of a concept map.** S: Lists three key points about the classmate and writes topic sentences and details for each paragraph.
Short-Term Goal: Composes a first draft	
7. Selects a variety of appropriate and meaningful key words related to the topic.	SLP: **Your assignment is to write about an angry lion. Try to use a variety of words to describe the lion. Think of words that are synonyms for the word *wild*.** S: **I could use the words *untamed, fierce,* and *ferocious*.**
8. Anticipates that the written work will require several drafts before it is complete.	SLP: **To write your best paper for school, you will make several drafts. What are some things you can do to be sure it's your best paper?** S: **Write "First Draft" on the draft or save it on a computer for ease in making edits to the second draft. Read each draft carefully for errors and to be sure my ideas are expressed concisely and clearly.**

Objectives	Examples
9. Organizes main ideas into topic sentences that contain a subject and an opinion.	SLP: **We just read the novel *A Wrinkle in Time*. Write a topic sentence for a paragraph about the main character.** S: (writes) Impatience was the primary motivating characteristic of Meg Murray, the main character.
10. Organizes paragraphs into main ideas and supporting details.	SLP: **When writing your paragraph, you will need a main idea and some details to support it.** S: Writes a topic sentence and lists three to four details to support it.
11. Provides a concluding statement or section or a sense of closure.	SLP: **The way you end your paper is just as important as the way you begin it. What should be included in your conclusion?** S: **The conclusion should (1) emphasize the importance of the thesis, (2) summarize the main ideas, (3) provide a sense of completeness, and (4) leave a final impression with the reader.**
12. Uses appropriate transition words, imagery, and tone.	SLP: **To make your writing interesting, you should use some transition words and imagery and decide on a certain tone. Tell me some of each of these, and then write one sentence for each type.** S: **Transition words are words like *since, so, after that, in the beginning, therefore*. Imagery means to use descriptions or metaphors. The tone could be friendly, serious, or funny.** (writes) Transition: The boy was tired, therefore he sat down under a shade tree. Imagery: The boiling hot sun was beating down on his back. Tone: Clean up this mess, and I mean this minute!
Short-Term Goal: Proofs the written work	
13. Recognizes and corrects spelling, punctuation, and capitalization.	SLP: **After writing the first draft of your narrative, use the C.O.P.S. acronym to proofread four times. What does C.O.P.S. mean?** S: **Capitalization, organization, punctuation, and spelling**
14. Recognizes and corrects errors in word content, grammar, and syntax.	SLP: **When you proofread the first draft of your report this time, check for correct verb tenses, pronoun antecedent agreement, sentence structure, and a variety of nouns and verbs.** S: Rereads the report, using a different colored pencil to correct each of the areas listed.

(*continues*)

Objectives	Examples
15. Recognizes and corrects inconsistencies or lack of coherence between sentences.	SLP: **When proofing a written social studies report, you need to make sure that your sentences flow logically and make sense.** S: Reads the paper to find inconsistencies between sentences, makes changes, and rereads until the text makes sense to the writer or another reader.
Short-Term Goal: Revises and edits the written work	
16. Revises the content to achieve clarity.	SLP: **With a partner, take turns reading your story to each other and decide whether it is clear and easy to follow.** S: Works with a partner to determine clarity of the story, and then rewrites the parts that are unclear.
17. Revises the content to achieve brevity.	SLP: **In writing, you want to be sure not to use extra words or sentences. With your partner, reread your stories. What are some things you should look for to delete?** S: **We could delete unnecessary words, phrases, or sentences or combine simple sentences to make compound or complex sentences.**
18. Revises the content for overall organization.	SLP: **Here are some things to remember when finalizing your book report. It should not be too long. It needs to be clear and well organized so that the reader truly understands what you have written. With your partner, read your book reports to each other.** S: Classmates trade papers and then report to each other on whether the content is clear and well organized.
19. Revises the content for use (e.g., pragmatics).	SLP: **You need to consider who will be reading what you write. Write a thank-you note to your friend, and then write a thank-you note to an adult. How are the two notes different?** S: Writes a thank-you note to a friend and to an adult. **The thank-you note to my friend is more casual, with words we might use when talking to each other. The one to the adult is more formal and respectful.**

Objectives	Examples
Short-Term Goal: Uses technology to publish the written work	
20. Makes the written piece into a final work to share with a variety of audiences.	SLP: **There are many ways to publish your written work so that others can read it. Publishing a work can be as simple as completing a neatly written copy to display on a bulletin board. You may also have it printed to submit to a literary magazine. How will you publish yours?** S: **My friends encouraged me when they read my poem. I would like to type a copy on the computer and submit it to the *Martin School Literary Magazine*.**
21. Accepts feedback received from the audience.	SLP: **You have heard feedback from your peers. As the author, how can you make your readers' feedback most beneficial to you?** S: **I can thank my friends and think about how I can use their ideas to improve my story and how to publish it.**
22. Revises and edits the written work based on constructive feedback from others.	SLP: **After reading a story to an audience, you must consider the comments from your audience about your story. How will you edit your work before submitting the story for the writing contest?** S: **I will edit the second paragraph to include a more complete description of the main character.**

Unit 9

Speech Production

- Traditional Articulation Approach
- Phonological Pattern Approach

Speech is the production of phonemes and includes articulated sounds and syllables. It is a part of the overall system of communication (Peña-Brooks & Hegde, 2000). *Speech* has been defined as "a system that relates meaning with sound" (Kent, 1998, p. 1). A *speech–sound disorder* can range from a disorder as mild as a lisp to a disorder such as that found in an individual who is completely unintelligible (Bernthal, Bankson, & Flipsen, 2013). Most speech–language pathologists (SLPs) working with children will have individuals with speech–sound disorders on their caseloads. A 2010 report from Mullen and Schooling indicated that up to 56% of the caseloads of school-based clinicians could involve work on speech–sound production.

The objectives in this unit are meant to facilitate planning for the treatment of these disorders. The objectives are divided into two sections: Traditional Articulation Approach and Phonological Pattern Approach. A thorough assessment of the student's speech production, which evaluates both specific phoneme errors and patterns of phoneme production, will help determine which approach is most appropriate for therapy. Many severely unintelligible children benefit from the phonological pattern approach and may move to the articulation approach at the point when only a few specific sound errors remain.

Traditional Articulation Approach

This approach emphasizes the proper positioning of the articulators (correct phonemic placement) and a variety of activities for remediation of the error sounds. The objectives in this section are presented in a developmental sequence to facilitate correct sound production. Although the objectives are presented sequentially, any of these objectives may be rearranged, omitted, or rewritten to suit an individual student's needs.

Phonological Pattern Approach

This approach is often suitable for children who have unintelligible speech. These students are delayed in using the appropriate phonological patterns expected for developing intelligible speech. According to Bishop and Adams (1990), unintelligible speech must be resolved by age 5 years 6 months to significantly reduce academic problems associated with speech disorders. The phonological pattern approach is based on the rules of the sound system of language that includes the set of phonemes and their permissible arrangement in oral language. Rather than focusing on the specific sound errors and correcting each one individually, this approach deals with deviant phonological patterns in the child's speech. Although there are different approaches used to treat phonological disorders, the objectives in this section have been adapted from the work of Barbara Hodson (2011).

Traditional Articulation Approach

Yearly Goal: *To produce speech sounds correctly in words in spontaneous speech*

Objectives	Examples
Short-Term Goal: Discriminates one sound from other sounds	
1. Listens to a group of isolated speech sounds and indicates when the target sound is heard.	SLP: **I'm going to say some different sounds. Raise your hand when you hear me say /f/.**
2. Indicates when the target sound is heard in words.	SLP: **I am going to say some words. Give me a thumbs up when you hear a word that starts with /f/.** S: Hears the word *fan* and shows a thumbs-up.
3. Indicates the position in which the target sound appears in words.	SLP: **Look at this train. It has an engine, a car, and a caboose. Now listen to me say some words with the /s/ sound. If you hear /s/ at the first of the word, touch the engine. If you hear /s/ in the middle of the word, touch the train car, and if /s/ is at the end of the word, touch the caboose.** S: Hears the word *kiss* and touches the train's caboose.
4. Indicates correct or incorrect production of the target sound in words spoken by the SLP.	SLP: **I'm going to name some pictures with the /r/ sound that we have been working on. If I say the /r/ sound correctly, put a block in the sack with the happy face. If the /r/ is not correct, put a block in the sack with the sad face.** S: Hears the word *run* articulated correctly and puts a block in the happy face sack.
5. Given two pictures that differ in only one sound in the initial or final position, points to the picture the SLP names (minimal pairs).	SLP: **Look at these two pictures. I will name both of them. Now listen carefully and put a sticker on the one that I say. This is a *wing*. This is a *ring*. Put your sticker on the ring.** S: Puts a sticker on the picture of a ring.
Short-Term Goal: Produces the sound in words	
6. Produces the target sound in isolation.	SLP: **Today we are going to learn the /f/ sound. I'll write in on the board. This is an *f* and it says /f/. Watch me bite my bottom lip and blow. Now you try it.** S: Watches SLP and attempts /f/ with modeling, shaping, and mirror work from the SLP as needed for correct production.

Objectives	Examples
7. Produces the target sound in syllables.	SLP: **We are going to play a game called Space Talk. All of the new words will start with your sound. This pencil is called *chee* in outer space talk. What are you holding? A book is called *cha*. What is your book?** S: **Chee, cha**
8. Produces the target sound in the initial word position.	SLP: **Look at these pictures on the floor that all begin with your special sound /k/. Each time you say /k/ correctly in a word, you can roll this car over it to the next picture. Let's see if you can make it all the way to the prize at the end of the road!** S: Says *key* with a good /k/ and rolls the car to the next picture. SLP: Provides modeling and feedback as needed for good /k/ production.
9. Produces the target sound in the final word position.	SLP: **All of these pictures on the wall have your special sound /s/ at the end. Let's turn off the light, and you can shine your flashlight on one of the pictures and name it. Be sure to say it with a good /s/ sound at the end of the word. What picture is your light on?** S: **Bus** SLP: Provides feedback and modeling as needed for a good /s/ production.
10. Produces the target sound in the medial word position.	SLP: **We are going to practice your /k/ sound when it is in the middle of words. Name the pictures that are taped on these blocks. They all have /k/ in the middle. Each time you say the word correctly, you can drop the block in the bucket.** S: After saying *pocket* correctly, drops the block in the bucket.
11. Produces the target sound in the initial, medial, and final word positions.	SLP: **Name these pictures. They all have your speech sound /f/ in the beginning, middle, or end. Now I will ask you some questions. Answer by pointing to the correct picture and saying the answer with a good /f/ sound. Let's try one. When you share an apple with someone, you each get one _____.** S: **Half**

(continues)

Objectives	Examples
12. Produces the target sound in consonant clusters in the initial word position.	SLP: **Look at these pictures, and let's name them. They start with your /s/ sound. Listen to my question and name and give me the correct picture. Which picture goes with a fork?** S: **Spoon**
13. Produces the target sound in consonant clusters in the final word position.	SLP: **In my special bag today are objects whose names end with your /s/ sound and another sound. Pull out an object and use your best /s/ to tell me what it is.** S: Pulls an object from the bag and says **mask**.
Short-Term Goal: Produces the sound in carrier phrases, phrases, and short sentences	
14. Produces the target sound in selected positions in words to complete a carrier phrase.	SLP: **Look at this sentence. It says, "I see a _____." I will read the sentence, and you can fill in the blank with the name of the card you draw from this pile. The names of the cards all have your /s/ sound at the end. Let's do one: "I see a _____."** S: **Mouse**
15. Produces the target sound in selected positions in words using carrier phrases.	SLP: **A pirate has hidden pictures with your /k/ sound at the end in this treasure box (a box full of beans). Dig in the treasure box and say "I found a _____" with the name of the picture you find.** S: Digs in the treasure box, finds a picture, and says **I found a lock.**
16. Produces the target sound in selected positions in words using phrases.	SLP: **I am going to hide some tokens around things that begin with your /r/ sound. When you find a token, use a phrase and a good /r/ to tell me where it is. Where is the blue token? Where is the red token?** S: **Under the rock, next to the ring**
17. Produces the target sound in selected positions in words in structured sentences.	SLP: **I have taped some pictures that have /s/ at the end on the wall. Let's name them. Now throw this beanbag at a picture, and use the word in a sentence. Be sure to say /s/ correctly at the end of the word.** S: Throws beanbag at the picture of a horse and says **I want to ride a horse.**

Objectives	Examples
18. Produces the target sound in selected positions in words when reading short sentences.	SLP: **I have written some sentences on these sentence strips. Find the picture that goes with each sentence. Now read that sentence with a good /l/ sound.** S: Matches the picture of lake to the sentence and reads **I see a boat on the lake.**
19. Produces the target sound in all word positions in sentences while playing a game.	SLP: **Let's play a game. Say your /r/ sound correctly every time you say these things: It's my turn. It's your turn. Roll the dice. I got three, or four.** S: Articulates /r/ correctly throughout the game.
20. Produces the target sound in all word positions while making up sentences about pictures.	SLP: **Look at this picture of a birthday party. There are lots of things at the party that have your /k/ and /g/ sounds. Let's name some of them: cake, candle, card, game, gift, guests, cookie, decorations, chocolate, napkin, bike, gift bag, like. Now use these words as you make up sentences about a birthday party with your best /k/ and /g/.** S: **I blew out the candles on my birthday cake. Guests brought gifts.**
21. Produces the target sound in all word positions in short responses to the SLP's questions.	SLP: **Answer my questions with a short sentence using your /l/ sound. What do we do at 1:00? What do you like to eat?** S: **We go to the library. I like to eat pizza.**
Short-Term Goal: Produces the sound in reading, describing pictures, telling stories, and spontaneous conversation	
22. Produces the target sound in all word positions while reading a paragraph.	SLP: **Look at this paragraph about our field trip to the zoo. First, underline all of the /r/ sounds. Now read the paragraph aloud with your best /r/.**
23. Produces the target sound in all word positions while describing pictures that tell a story.	SLP: **These pictures tell a story about a trip to the grocery store. Put them in order, and use your good /s/ sound as you tell the story.** S: **We drove to the store. We bought some carrots. We put them in a sack.**
24. Produces the target sound in all word positions in sentences while telling a story.	SLP: **Do you know the story of *Pancakes for Breakfast*? Let's make a list and practice saying some words in that story that have your speech sound. Now tell me the story using your best speech. I will put a check mark by each of the words in our list that you use and say correctly.**

(continues)

Objectives	Examples
25. Produces the target sound in all word positions in sentences while role playing.	SLP: **Let's pretend that we are going on a camping trip. What are some /r/ words that we can use when talking about our camping trip?** S: **river, rain, rocky, forest, arrow, bear, campfire, star** SLP: **Practice saying those words correctly, and then we can use them as we pretend to go camping.** S: **We camped by a river and built a campfire.**
26. Produces the target sound in all positions in words in spontaneous conversation with a peer in the speech room for 3 minutes.	SLP: **While you and Jennifer are talking about what you are going to do after school today, I will be listening for good production of your speech sounds.**
27. Produces the target sound in all positions in words in spontaneous conversation outside the speech room with a parent, teacher, or friend for 5 minutes.	SLP: **I am going to ask your parents to listen for your /r/ sound as you talk on the way home from school today or at dinner tonight. I hope you say them all correctly!**

Phonological Pattern Approach

Yearly Goal: *To increase intelligibility by suppressing exhibited phonological patterns*

Note: Only those patterns that are consistently deficient and stimulable should be targeted.

Objectives	Examples
Short-Term Goal: Suppresses use of primary target patterns	
1. Suppresses the pattern of *syllable reduction* (a reduced number of syllables in the production of a word or utterance: *pop* for *popcorn*) and replaces it with the production of two- and three-syllable words. *Note:* Productions are correct as long as there is a vowel for each syllable, even if parts of the rest of the word are omitted or misarticulated.	SLP: Models multisyllabic names of toys while playing with the child. **"Bubbles." Let's blow bubbles. Again? Say "bubbles." This is a banana. Would you like it? Say "banana."** S: Names *bubbles* and *banana*, marking all syllables.
2. Suppresses the pattern of *initial consonant deletion* (absence of single consonants at the beginning of words: *at* for *hat*) and replaces it with the production of initial consonants in words.	SLP: Takes objects that represent one-syllable words beginning with a single consonant sound out of a grab bag and names them. **This is a ball. Say *ball*. This is a mouse. Say *mouse*.** S: Repeats names of toys. SLP: Emphasizes the initial consonant by elongating or increasing volume and repeating models until the child articulates the initial consonant with the rest of the word.

Objectives	Examples
3. Suppresses the pattern of *final consonant deletion* (omission of single consonants at the end of words: *ca* for *cat*) and replaces it with the production of final consonants in words.	SLP: **Stand up against this paper I have on the wall, and I will trace your body. Now let's name the parts. Be sure to put a sound on the end of the word: *nose, leg, head, arm, eyes, neck, lip, foot*.** S: Repeats names of CVC body parts. SLP: Emphasizes final consonants and provides models as needed.
4. Suppresses the pattern of *velar fronting* (substitution of alveolar sounds for velar sounds: *teep* for *keep*) and replaces it with correct production of velars in words. *Note:* Velars should be presented in this order: final /k/, initial /k/, initial /g/.	SLP: **I have drawn some bugs on the board and taped pictures of your /k/ and /g/ sounds below them. Take this flyswatter and swat one of the bugs. Then name the picture you swatted with your best speech.** S: Swats bugs on the board and names one syllable words such as *car*, *key*, *go*, and *gum* with good velar sounds.
5. Suppresses the pattern of *backing* (front sounds are replaced by back sounds) and replaces it with correct production of alveolar sounds in words. *Note:* Alveolar sounds are the sounds most frequently backed: *cap* for *tap*, *hun* for *sun*.	SLP: **Let's go fishing for picture cards of one-syllable words that begin with your speech sounds. Remember to start these words in the front of your mouth. What did you catch?** S: **Top, soup**
6. Suppresses the pattern of */s/ cluster reduction* (omitting the /s/ phoneme in a consonant cluster: *poon* for *spoon*) and replaces it with correct production of /s/ clusters in words.	SLP: **Let's decorate cookies while working on your /s/ sound. First, repeat these words after me that we will use while we decorate: *spoon, stove, stir, smell, spread, sprinkles*. Be sure to say the /s/ sound on these words while we decorate the cookies.** S: **Let's use this spoon to stir the icing. I want lots of sprinkles on my cookie.**
7. Suppresses the pattern of *liquid gliding* (replacing a liquid sound with a glide: *wake* for *lake*) and replaces it with correct production of initial /l/ or /r/. *Note:* Initial /l/ and /r/ clusters are additional possible targets at this stage.	SLP: **Look at these laminated pictures in the bottom of this plastic container. They all start with /r/. Sprinkle some "rain" on a picture, then name it with your best /r/ sound.** S: Repeats the names of all of the pictures after the SLP's model. Then, using a spray bottle, squirts water on each picture before naming it. Says these words: ***rain*, *rock*, *rope*, *run*, *rabbit*, *robin*, *rainbow*, *raft*.**

(continues)

Objectives	Examples
Short-Term Goal: Suppresses use of secondary potential target patterns *Note:* These patterns should be considered if they are still present after the student has demonstrated acquisition of the primary target patterns.	
8. Suppresses the pattern of *prevocalic voicing* (replacing a voiceless prevocalic consonant with a voiced sound: *gate* for *Kate*) and replaces it with correct production of word initial voiceless consonants.	SLP: While playing with minimal-pair picture cards whose feature is initial voicing: **Look at these two pictures: *gold, cold*. Put a block on the picture of *cold*. Say *cold*. Now you can use the block to start building a tower. Let's do another one: *Kate, gate*. Put a block on *Kate* and say it. Now add to your tower.** S: Adds a block to the tower with each correct response.
9. Suppresses the pattern of *vowel neutralization* (reducing most vowels to /ʌ/ or /ɑ/: *mutt* for *mitt* and *mat*) and replaces it with correct production of vowels in words.	SLP: **Each time you say the name of one of these pictures correctly, you will win a puzzle piece. Let's see if you can complete the puzzle.** S: **Can, bat, ship, pill**
10. Suppresses the pattern of *stridency deletion* (omitting the stridency feature by substituting a nonstrident sound or by omitting the sound: *pour* for *four*) and replaces it with the correct production of strident sounds, especially /s/ and /f/, in words.	SLP: **Let's name these /s/ and /f/ pictures and then put them into things at home and things at school. Now use the names of these pictures to answer my questions. Use your best speech. (1) What can be around the backyard? (2) What do we do in music class? (3) What is in your refrigerator at home? (4) What brings children to school?** S: **(1) fence, (2) sing, (3) food, (4) bus**
11. Suppresses the pattern of *depalitalization* (palatal component is deleted from a palatal phoneme: *sew* for *show*) and replaces it with correct production of a palatal consonant: /ʃ, ʧ, ʤ/, and /ʒ/.	SLP: **Look at these seashells. There is a picture under each one of them. Pick up a shell and put it in your bucket. Then name the picture with your best speech.** S: Picks up shells and names pictures such as *shell*, *chair*, *jump*, and *measure*.
12. Suppresses the pattern of *additional consonant cluster reduction* (omitting a consonant in clusters containing glides such as *qu*, *few*; some medial and final clusters in words such as *boxing* and *best*; and three-consonant clusters as in the words *splash* and *sixth*) and replaces it with correct production of all consonant clusters.	SLP: **Every time you name one of these pictures with good speech, you will get a piece to make this clown face craft. Let's see if you can finish his funny face!** S: Earns a piece of the craft while saying words such as *beauty*, *music*, *mixing*, *first*, *straight*, and *sixth*.
13. Suppresses the pattern of *postvocalic syllabic vowelization* (replacing a postvocalic or syllabic liquid with a vowel like *u* or *o*: *tabo* for *table*) and replaces it with correct production of postvocalic syllabic /r/ and /l/ in words.	SLP: **Look at this picture of a house. It has some things and people that have your speech sounds. Let's name those pictures with good speech, and then use them to answer my questions. What do you see in the kitchen? Who is in the living room?** S: **Apple, table, waffle; mother, grandfather**

Objectives	Examples
14. Suppresses the pattern of *assimilation* (altering a phoneme so that it takes on a characteristic of another sound in the word: *lello* for *yellow*, *kruck* for *truck*) and replaces it with correct production of the targeted phoneme in words.	SLP: **We are going to mail your special words. Say the word with your best speech, tell me whom you are mailing it to, and then put it in the mailbox.** Words are ones that the student typically assimilates. S: **Yellow. I'm mailing it to Mom.** **Coat. I'm mailing it to my brother.**

Unit 10

Voice

- **Modification of the Speaking Environment**
- **Knowledge of Vocal Structures and Voice Production**
- **Recognition and Elimination of Vocal Abuse Behaviors**
- **Voice Quality Improvement**
- **Transfer and Maintenance**

The most common cause for voice problems in school-age children referred to speech–language pathologists (SLPs) is hoarseness related to hyperfunctional misuse of the voice (Boone, McFarlane, Von Berg, & Zraick, 2010, p. 182). Endoscopy in these children will reveal vocal fold thickening or vocal nodules or polyps (Boone et al., 2010, p. 182). Providing voice therapy for children who present with vocal nodules that result in voice disorders is important. They do not simply "outgrow" the problem. Even after surgical treatment for symptoms of abuse, better use of the voice is necessary to maintain improved voice quality (Justice, 2010, p. 388).

For students to acquire and maintain a healthy voice, it is important for them to achieve these overall goals: (a) Show concern about a voice disorder before beginning voice therapy, (b) reduce the vocal abuses and alter the speaking environment that led to the physical changes in the vocal structure, (c) understand the vocal structures and mechanics of voice production, (d) recognize and eliminate vocal abuse behaviors, (e) learn a healthy manner of voice production, and (f) transfer and maintain improved voice production to all speaking situations. Transfer occurs at all levels.

Students with voice disorders require the collaborative efforts of many people. Boone et al. (2010) reported studies that indicate that children with "vocal nodules often require strong psychological support by the voice clinician" (p. 125). When medical personnel, SLPs, teachers, parents, and other family members work together, the outlook for a positive result to voice therapy is highly increased. Referring physicians are crucial to the team effort when vocal abuse is identified as the causative factor in medical diagnosis of vocal nodules, polyps, and contact ulcers. Equally important is the role of the student. The student must take active responsibility for vocal practices. The objectives in this unit give the student responsibility to practice new vocal skills as guided by the SLP, supported by the physician's diagnosis and checkups, and assisted by parents at home and teachers in the school setting.

Description of Contents

The objectives in this unit provide examples of situations in which students practice a voice goal within a small-group setting, such as a speech class, with the SLP's support, because independent practice outside that setting is not yet appropriate. The school setting is often an excellent place to practice alternative vocal habits and use of the new, clear voice during transfer throughout therapy. These voice objectives are most useful for students who are age 6 years or older.

Modification of the Speaking Environment. The objectives in this section are designed for the student, siblings, parents, and teachers. The SLP provides information to the student, parents, and teachers to help them work together to develop an atmosphere that supports learning to use a healthy voice. It is generally considered optimal, at this point, for the student to show evidence of concern about the voice disorder and a desire to enter into treatment.

Knowledge of Vocal Structures and Voice Production. These objectives assist the SLP when planning to teach voice terminology, mechanics of voice production, and the structure and processes of the vocal mechanism. When students learn to explain normal voice production, it helps them develop an objective attitude toward the voice disorder. It also increases understanding of the need to eliminate vocally abusive behaviors and replace them with healthy vocal habits.

Recognition and Elimination of Vocal Abuse Behaviors. This set of objectives is designed to help the students identify vocal abuse in general without focusing on the students' own vocal abuse behaviors. Objectives advance to those that help them identify their own abusive voice habits and, finally, to those where students eliminate their own vocally abusive habits one at a time.

Voice Quality Improvement. These objectives focus on releasing extraneous muscular tension in the head and neck area, learning appropriate breath control, and producing a clear voice quality. SLPs may choose to begin objectives in this section before completing the objectives in the third section. These objectives can be adapted to their own successful voice intervention methods.

Transfer and Maintenance. The transfer and maintenance objectives are useful throughout voice therapy, not just toward the end of therapy. That is because students need to gradually transfer their newly learned healthy voice to speaking situations outside the therapy room. The same is true of the elimination of vocal abuse. Transfer of improved voice quality and elimination of vocal abuse occurs throughout the therapy process.

Modification of the Speaking Environment

Yearly Goal: *To modify the speaking environment to assist in achieving healthy vocal care and voice quality that is clear, has appropriate loudness and pitch, and is free from vocal tension in all speaking situations*

Objectives	Examples
1. Develops an environment conducive to optimal voice production.	SLP: **When you and I met with your family, we talked about ways to make your household a quieter place where it's easier for everyone to use a healthy voice. What did your family decide to do?** S: **We'll start turning down the TV instead of trying to talk over it. If no one is watching TV, we'll turn it off. We'll play music at a lower volume. Instead of talking over them, we will turn off loud appliances, such as blenders and hair dryers, before talking to each other.**
2. Discusses new ways to modify the general speaking behavior in the family.	SLP: **During our meeting with your family, we talked about ways your family plans to lower the loudness level of speaking in your house. Let's talk about the plan, and I'll write it down.** S: **We'll walk up to each other when we want to talk instead of yelling through the house. We'll get each other's attention before beginning a conversation. Everyone will lower the volume on our headphones so we're not tempted to talk loudly over them. We can take turns talking instead of all talking at once.**
3. Applies understanding of the harmful effects of yelling.	SLP: **What happens when you clap your hands together hard and fast for a long time? Yes, they get red and sore. What do you think happens to the vocal folds when they are banged together?** S: **They become red and sore.**
4. Applies knowledge about the harmful effects of talking against background noise.	SLP: **Background noise makes it tempting to shout to be heard. Where are some places you go where there's background noise? What can you and your family members do about it? When you and I met with your parents yesterday, we talked about ways to stop talking over loud noise. What are the things your family plans to do?** S: **We will walk up to each other to talk instead of yelling through the house. Instead of playing music loudly, we'll turn it down.**

(continues)

Objectives	Examples
5. Applies knowledge of the harmful effects of hard throat clearing and habitual coughing.	SLP: **You can damage your vocal cords by hard throat clearing and lots of coughing. I want you to start drinking sips of water during the day to help you avoid coughing. Let's talk about ways you can drink more water during the day.** S: **I can get permission from my teachers to keep a bottle of water with me at school. I can also stop at a water fountain between classes.**
6. Applies knowledge of the harmful effects of loud singing.	SLP: **Your doctor who examined your vocal cords gave the order not to sing at school until you've learned new ways to produce your voice. Your teachers and principal have approved the restriction. How do you feel about that?** S: **It shows me that it's important to work hard to change the way I use my voice. I take it seriously.**
7. Applies knowledge of the harmful effects of a very dry atmosphere and takes steps to improve the situation with humidifiers or by providing opportunities to drink more water and juices.	SLP: **A very dry atmosphere is harmful to your vocal cords. What could you and your parents do to add humidity to your house?** S: **We could put a humidifier in my bedroom.**
8. Applies knowledge of the harmful effects of very hot or spicy foods if determined to have an aggravating effect, such as frequent gastric reflux.	SLP: **The doctor has determined that eating very spicy foods has led to your gastric reflux. Your diet will need to be modified. How do you feel about that?** S: **I'm willing to follow the doctor's instructions about the foods I eat. It's important.**
9. Maintains a period of vocal rest if indicated by the physician's laryngological report.	SLP: **Your vocal folds are quite damaged. Your doctor has recommended that you not speak at all for a very short time. How are ways you can communicate without using your voice?** S: **I can write notes or use gestures.**
10. Shows concern about the voice disorder before beginning the voice improvement program after learning about the results of vocal abuse from the physician and SLP.	SLP: **Now that you understand the results of vocal abuse on your vocal folds, what do you think about starting therapy to learn how to have a healthy voice?** S: **It bothers me a lot that I've injured my vocal cords with loud talking and yelling. I want to start learning how to take care of my voice right away.**

Knowledge of Vocal Structures and Voice Production

Yearly Goal: *To demonstrate knowledge of the structures and functions of the respiratory tract and how the voice is produced*

Objectives	Examples
1. Given a picture or line drawing of the respiratory tract, describes and traces the pathway for respiration and speaking, and points to and explains pictures to show a basic understanding of phonation and the structure and function of the vocal mechanism.	SLP: **We don't usually think about how we breathe or talk, but today we're going to take time to describe the process of respiration and your respiratory tract. Look at your picture of a person's upper body and point to each part that I name. Then say its name.** S: (points to and names) **nose, mouth, pharynx, larynx, trachea, bronchi, lungs, bronchial tree, air sacs, diaphragm**
2. Using a picture of the respiratory tract, traces the inhalation pathway.	SLP: **Complete my sentences as you trace the inhalation pathway. You take in air through your _____. The air continues down your _____ and through your _____ and into your _____. As your lungs fill with air, they push against your _____ so that they expand.** S: **mouth or nose, throat, windpipe or trachea, lungs, ribs**
3. Following the SLP's demonstration and instruction, produces humming and single words on exhalation.	SLP: **When you have used the air you breathed in, it travels back up the same pathway it came down. Let's feel what happens when the air comes in, fills the lungs, and goes out. Place your left hand around your body to feel your right ribs and take a breath. Do you feel your ribs moving outward and inward with each breath? Now I want you to hum (hmmmm) and let your breath carry the sound out through your nose. Now say "hi."** S: **Hmmm. Hi.**
4. Shows knowledge of the vocabulary that deals with vocal hygiene (e.g., vocal abuse, phonation, vocal folds, lungs, larynx).	SLP: **Last week we talked about proper care of our voices. Now choose a word on the board to finish these sentences: Using your voice in a harsh way that can harm it is called _____. Creating sound with your voice is called _____. The valve inside the larynx that opens and closes to create sound is called the _____. When you breathe in, the air fills up the _____.** S: **Vocal abuse, phonation, vocal cords, lungs**

(continues)

Objectives	Examples
5. Understands and explains the changes in vocal cords that result from vocal abuse.	SLP: **Let's look at this picture of the respiratory tract and the vocal cords and talk about what vocal abuse does to vocal cords. When they are healthy, vocal cords close together smoothly. Your vocal cords hit together very hard when you yell, scream, use a loud voice, make motor or animal sounds, or cry loudly. What will happen if you do that too much?** S: **My vocal cords could get red and swollen and possibly form a small nodule.**

Recognition and Elimination of Vocal Abuse Behaviors

Yearly Goal: *To recognize and eliminate vocal abuse behaviors*

Objectives	Examples
Short-Term Goal: Identifies vocal abuse behaviors in situations that promote either vocal abuse or good vocal hygiene behaviors without focusing directly on own personal vocal abuse behaviors	
1. Identifies pictures that show situations of vocal abuse.	SLP: **Look at these pictures of people. Some of them are abusing their voices, and others are using their voices correctly. Circle the pictures that show vocal abuse.** S: Circles pictures of a man yelling and a child making motor sounds while playing with a car.
2. Describes and discusses situations of vocal abuse in others.	SLP: **Listen for vocal abuse in this recording. Raise your hand when you hear it and then describe it.** S: Indicates when she hears vocal abuse and describes it as *yelling*, *hard throat clearing*, *talking over noise*, *imitating vehicle sounds*, and *loud laughing*.
3. Identifies situations and settings that promote vocal abuse.	SLP: **Look at this list of speaking situations. We will write "yes" by the ones that might cause vocal abuse and "no" by those that do not.** S: **Yes: Talking over loud music, talking in a voice too high or too low, talking too long on the phone, clearing the throat too often. No: Talking to a friend next to you in a quiet room, answering your teacher's question in class, talking with a friend in your healthy voice while on a walk.**

Objectives	Examples
4. Demonstrates knowledge of the situations where vocal abuse and misuse may occur.	SLP: **Look at these pictures. Arrange them to show the easiest to most difficult for using a good voice.** S: Arranges pictures in this order: talking to a friend on the phone, ordering at a fast food restaurant, cheering at a football game.
5. Identifies healthy voice alternatives to vocal abuse in situations that might encourage vocal abuse.	SLP: **Look at these two columns. One has a list of situations that could cause vocal abuse and one has healthy alternatives. Draw lines to match the healthy practice that could replace the vocal abuse.** S: Draws lines to match: yelling and waving, loud cheering and clapping, talking at a loud concert and talking in a quiet place.
Short-Term Goal: Eliminates own identified vocal abuses by targeting one abuse at a time	
6. Hierarchically lists situations where own vocal abuse occurs.	SLP: **Think about the situations in which you have vocal abuse. Now number and list them from the easiest to the most difficult for you to use a healthy voice.** S: **(1) Talking to my friend on the playground. (2) Running with my dad. (3) Cheering for the soccer team.**
7. Identifies and keeps track of own vocal abuse and healthy voice use.	SLP: **To reduce unhealthy use of your voice, you need to become aware of it. On this note card, write down or draw pictures of some ways you abuse your voice. Pay attention to your voice today and put an *X* beside the picture description when you notice yourself using that kind of vocal abuse. Bring it back the next time I see you, and we will discuss the results.**
8. Identifies personal healthy voice alternatives to vocal abuse.	SLP: **Write down two ways you have vocal abuse and healthy voice alternatives. Try to use the healthy choices this week.** S: (writes) (1) Instead of yelling so loudly at the game, I will try to remember to clap and stomp my feet. (2) Instead of clearing my throat, I'll sip water.

Voice Quality Improvement

Yearly Goal: *To improve voice quality*

Objectives	Examples
Short-Term Goal: Eliminates extraneous muscular tension and develops appropriate breath support	
1. Identifies vocal and associated muscular tension.	SLP: **We've just watched scenes from a TV show where people yell or talk with too much force. Let's talk about what you saw people doing when talking while they were tense.** S: **A woman tightened her face and neck muscles. A boy clenched his fists. A cheerleader looked tense when she yelled.**
2. Imitates and demonstrates progressive relaxation.	SLP: **Follow my lead as we do these progressive relaxation exercises. We'll begin by moving the large muscle groups in the legs and arms. Finally, we'll work to release the tension in the muscles of the head and neck area.** S: Imitates exercises as demonstrated by the SLP.
3. Describes and imitates central breathing and breath control.	SLP: **With your speech partner, describe and imitate optimal breath support for speaking (central breathing).** S: **Your abdomen and rib cage expand when you take a breath in. The shoulders do not rise because your expanded abdomen and rib cage allow the lungs to fill up without raising the shoulders. Raising the shoulders would create tension. When you begin to speak, your abdomen and rib cage return to the first position as the air is used in tiny puffs for speaking.**
4. Adds phonation while using central breathing.	SLP: **While practicing central breathing, add a gentle /h/ sound on exhalation. Good. Now add a vowel sound to the /h/: *hah, hoo, hi, hoe, he*. Good! We will gradually increase the length of your phonation to words, phrases, and sentences.** S: **/h/: *hah, hoo, hi, hoe, he***
5. Produces clear vowel sounds during central breathing after releasing muscular tension.	SLP: **With your partner, guide each other through your progressive relaxation exercises. Now say words to each other that begin with /h/. As you energize your voice from your abdominal area, "tie on" these vowel sounds: *a-e, o-e, ee, i-e, ih, ah, eh*. Now say these words that begin with vowels: *I'm, out, eel, ace, ice, owl*.** S: **(1) *a-e, o-e, ee, i-e, ih, ah, eh*. (2) I'm, out, eel, ace, ice, owl.**

Objectives	Examples
6. Produces clear, relaxed words and phrases while participating in the chewing technique.	SLP: **Today we'll begin with upper body release exercises. Then we'll use the chewing technique with single words and phrases while we sit in front of the mirror. Keep on saying clear but relaxed words and phrases. Now I'll ask you some questions as I chew. You answer as you "chew" your words: My speech is sloppy. Is your speech sloppy? What are you doing?** S: (while chewing) **I'm chewing. My speech is sloppy!**
7. Discriminates the old voice from the new healthy voice (relaxed, with appropriate breath flow, and optimal pitch).	SLP: **Today we'll record your voice first as you read a short paragraph. Then we'll record you while talking. When we listen to the recording, raise your hand when you hear your healthy voice.** S: Raises hand when hearing his or her healthy voice on the recording.
Short-Term Goal: Produces a clear voice quality following soft glottal-attack after instruction	
8. Uses soft glottal-attack voice following a yawn-sigh.	SLP: **Yawning helps you learn to say syllables and words starting with /h/ with a relaxed, easy voice. Let's try some.** S: Yawn-"**huh,**" yawn-"**hah,**" yawn-"**hum**"
9. Uses a soft glottal-attack voice in syllables beginning with /h/.	SLP: **Listen to these syllables that begin with /h/. Repeat them after me with a soft glottal-attack voice.** S: (repeats syllables such as) **hah, hih, huh**
10. Uses a soft glottal-attack voice in one-syllable /h/ words.	SLP: **Reach into this hat, pull out a word that starts with /h/, and say it after me with a soft glottal-attack voice.** S: (repeats) **hull, hum, hug**
11. Uses a soft glottal-attack voice in two-syllable /h/ words.	SLP: **Repeat one of my two-syllable /h/ words with a soft glottal-attack voice.** S: (repeats words such as) **honey, happy, hammock**
12. Uses a soft glottal-attack voice in three-syllable /h/ words or phrases.	SLP: **Each time you repeat after me one of these three-syllable words or phrases that start with /h/ with your soft glottal-attack voice, you will win a cotton ball. Glue them on this page to make a snowman.** S: (repeats) **honeydew, holiday, hurry up**

(continues)

Objectives	Examples
13. Uses a soft glottal-attack voice in four-syllable sentences beginning with /h/.	SLP: **Let's play Flashlight Tag. There are cards with four-syllable sentences that begin with the /h/ sound taped on the walls. When I turn the lights off, shine your flashlight on one of them. Then repeat it after me with a soft voice.** S: (repeats after SLP) **Who had hiccups?**
14. Uses a soft glottal-attack voice in six-syllable sentences initiated by /h/.	SLP: **There are sentences with six syllables taped on the wall. They all begin with the /h/ sound. Hit one with this beanbag, and then repeat it after me with a soft voice.** S: (repeats this sentence) **He hardly heard Harvey.**
15. Uses a soft glottal-attack voice in eight-syllable sentences.	SLP: **I am going to say some sentences that have eight syllables. Repeat them after me using a soft glottal-attack voice. Try this one: Have you ever been so hungry?** S: Repeats the sentence with a soft glottal-attack voice.
16. Uses a soft glottal-attack voice to finish a carrier phrase with a three- or four-syllable /h/ word.	SLP: **I want you to practice using a soft glottal-attack voice to finish this carrier phrase with a multisyllable /h/ word: Have Tom whisper _____.** S: **Have Tom whisper ______. (1) Hermione, (2) holiday, (3) helicopter**
17. Uses a clear, relaxed voice to say sentences of varied numbers of syllables.	SLP: **We are going to practice using a clear, relaxed voice while reading some sentences. Read these sentences with a soft glottal-attack: Harry is hard at work on his hobby. His hat is high.** S: Repeats sentences with a soft glottal-attack.
18. Uses a clear, relaxed voice while reading aloud.	SLP: **Let's practice reading aloud from your reader before you are asked to do it in class. Be sure to use a soft voice.** S: Reads aloud with a relaxed voice.

Transfer and Maintenance

Yearly Goal: *To transfer improved voice quality to environments outside the treatment setting and maintain elimination of vocal misuse and abuse*

Objectives	Examples
1. Consistently maintains complete elimination of vocal misuse and abuse.	SLP: **I want you to chart times of vocal misuse or abuse. You will keep doing this until there have been no instances for 2 weeks. Then, your healthy voice practices will be a habit.**

Objectives	Examples
2. Uses the new clear, healthy voice during conversations in speech class for increasingly longer periods of time.	SLP: **When talking with a friend or with me in speech class, use your new voice while you talk. We'll gradually increase the talking time from 5 minutes to about 20 minutes.**
3. Uses the new clear, healthy voice during conversations with family and peers for increasingly longer periods of time.	SLP: **Now that you are using your clear, healthy voice with me, it is time to start using it with your friends and family. Keep a chart each day, and write down some times that you used your best voice with your friends at school and with your family at home. We will talk about your chart next week.** S: Brings chart to speech class to discuss with SLP.
4. Maintains and monitors use of the new clear, healthy voice for progressively longer periods of time before dismissal (e.g., 1 week, 2 weeks, a month).	SLP: **Because of your good progress, you'll need to come to speech class only once after a week, then after 2 weeks, and then after a month. After that, if are still using your healthy voice, you'll be finished!**
5. Independently uses information and strategies for healthy voice use and care and handles any relapses after dismissal from formal voice treatment.	SLP: **After you are dismissed from voice therapy, what can you do if you begin to notice an increase in vocal misuse, abuse, or harsh voice quality?** S: **I can figure out what is causing the voice problems and replace that cause with strategies I have learned.**
6. If unable to handle a relapse, makes contact for "refresher" treatment.	SLP: **What will you do if you are not able to handle a relapse in your voice on your own?** S: **I will contact you or tell my parents or classroom teacher about the need for help to regain a healthy voice.**

Unit 11

Fluency

- Modification of the Communication Environment
- Young Children and Individuals With Less Advanced Stuttering
- Older Students and Individuals With More Advanced Stuttering
- Maintenance and Transfer of Improved Fluency

When stuttering hinders a student's ability to communicate, life at school and home is altered. Stuttering can interfere with the student's relationships with peers and participation in the classroom. Your responsibility as the speech–language pathologist (SLP) is to help the student become more fluent and, in doing so, increase the student's chances for personal and academic success.

Currently, methods and approaches for stuttering intervention abound. The objectives presented in this unit do not offer yet another technique. Instead, they serve as a general guide for planning therapy. The sections in this unit should be blended and recycled as the student makes progress. You are encouraged to take your own clinical expertise and successful intervention approaches into account when using these objectives to plan therapy.

The fluency intervention objectives will help students incorporate what has been learned during fluency activities into the "real world" of both the school day and social activities. This transfer is done by asking the student to do such things as list the speaking situations conducive to fluent speech, and chart stuttered and fluent speech during the school day. When the teachers, the family members, the student, and you all take a responsible part in therapy, the resulting boost to the student's motivation and program continuity increases the opportunities to reach the goal of more fluent speech production. Thus, social development and educational success are enhanced.

Description of Contents

This unit is divided into four parts: Modification of the Communication Environment, Young Children and Individuals With Less Advanced Stuttering, Older Students and Individuals With More Advanced Stuttering, and Maintenance and Transfer of Improved Fluency. The intervention objectives give examples of situations in which students are able to practice a fluency goal within a small-group setting, such as a speech class, with the support of the SLP, because independent practice in the classroom or outside that setting is not yet appropriate. The classroom is often an excellent place for practicing transfer that occurs throughout therapy. There are two sections of transfer objectives, one at the end of the objectives for Young Children and Individuals With Less Advanced Stuttering and one at the conclusion of Older Students and Individuals With More Advanced Stuttering.

Modification of the Communication Environment. The objectives in this section apply to individuals of all ages and with various levels of stuttering. These objectives are designed for the student, parents, siblings, teachers, and significant friends to work together to develop an atmosphere conducive to fluency. The objectives target fostering conditions that will encourage fluent speech. Appendix G contains lists of fluency facilitators that may be helpful with the objectives in this section.

Young Children and Individuals With Less Advanced Stuttering. The objectives in this section are designed to help them develop a more fluent manner of speaking and to transfer the achieved level of fluency to other locations and situations.

Older Students and Individuals With More Advanced Stuttering. The first part of this section contains objectives for helping students modify cognitive and affective behaviors that often interfere with long-term maintenance of improved fluency. The second part addresses development of an easier manner of stuttering. The third part contains objectives to help students develop a more fluent manner of speaking.

Maintenance and Transfer of Improved Fluency. Please refer to the objectives in this section for transfer during all stages of intervention. These objectives are designed to help students transfer improved fluency and an easier manner of stuttering to other environments from the beginning of intervention. Objectives for maintenance of improved fluency at the conclusion of intervention are also provided.

Modification of the Communication Environment

Yearly Goal: *To develop an atmosphere conducive to fluency*

Note: See Appendix G ("Fluency Facilitators") for help in planning intervention with the following objectives.

Objectives	Examples
1. Understands and implements with assistance ways to discuss the problem of stuttering openly in a "no big deal" manner.	SLP to parent: **If your child fell off her bicycle and was hurt, you would not ignore it. You would respond to how she felt. It's the same with stuttering. You need to acknowledge it and empathize with and respond to how your child feels about it. You could say something like "I noticed you had a hard time getting that word out, and that's okay."**
2. Allows the individual who stutters to "own" the problem of stuttering by allowing him or her to handle individual speaking situations and choose when to use "controls and tools," and by not allowing him or her to avoid speaking situations.	SLP to parent: **An important role in dealing with your child's speech is to encourage him to follow through with speaking situations instead of avoiding them. If your child has an upcoming presentation in class, let him know that it is his job to do it. Suggest that he discuss the presentation with his SLP, and together they can practice ways to make it a more successful experience.**
3. Rewards the courage and risk-taking in speaking activities in the individual who stutters.	SLP to parent and/or teacher: **Your child needs to know that her courage in taking part in speaking activities is noticed. Comments such as these will be helpful and encouraging :"I'm proud of you for going to the party yesterday and talking to some of your friends" or "You have been doing a great job lately of raising your hand and answering questions in class."**

Young Children and Individuals With Less Advanced Stuttering

Yearly Goal: *To communicate effectively in all speaking situations by using strategies that will enhance fluency and make stuttering easier*

Objectives	Examples
Short-Term Goal: Improves overall communication abilities by developing a more fluent manner of speaking	
1. Understands and applies the concepts of fast and slow in nonspeech and speech tasks.	SLP: **Look at this toy rabbit and turtle. Let's make the rabbit run fast. Now make the turtle crawl slowly. Today we're going to talk like rabbits and turtles. How would a rabbit talk? How would a turtle talk? When you hear me talk fast, point to the rabbit. When you hear me talk slow, point to the turtle. Now it's your turn. Let's practice saying "Twinkle, Twinkle, Little Star." When I point to the rabbit, say it fast, and when I point to the turtle, say it slowly.** S: **Fast. Slow.** Student says the poem with fast speech like the rabbit and then with slow speech like the turtle.
2. Understands and applies the concepts of smooth and bumpy (or sticky) in nonspeech and speech tasks.	SLP: **Sometimes our speech is bumpy, and sometimes it is smooth. I have glued some popcorn kernels on paper. Run your finger over them. Do they feel smooth or bumpy? Now listen to me count to five.** (Counts with repetitions.) **Was that smooth or bumpy?** S: **Bumpy** SLP: **Now run your finger along this table. Does it feel smooth or bumpy?** S: **Smooth** SLP: **See if you can imitate my smooth and bumpy speech as I count to five.**
3. Understands and applies the concepts of soft and loud in nonspeech and speech tasks.	SLP: **Today we are going to talk about soft and loud with this toy drum. First, play the drum softly. Now count to three in a soft voice. This time, beat on the drum loudly. Count to three in a loud voice.** S: Demonstrates understanding of soft and loud with the drum and with his voice.

Objectives	Examples
4. Understands and uses the communication skills of eye contact, listening, and turn taking.	SLP: **While we play Candy Land, we are going to practice being good speakers and listeners. These pictures will remind us of what to do: (1) eyes, (2) ears, (3) a person pointing to herself. Tell me what each of these means, and we will use them during our game.** S: **(1) Eyes: Look at the person you are talking to. (2) Ears: When you are not talking, it is your turn to listen to the person who is talking. (3) Person pointing to herself: This means sometimes it is my turn and sometimes it is your turn.**
5. Understands and uses the communication skill of phrasing.	SLP: **We are going to learn to put some pauses in our speech. As we play Go Fish, use pauses such as the following: It's / your turn. Do you have / a cowboy? You need to / Go Fish.**
6. Produces slow, smooth (easy) speech in quiet settings using structured tasks in which the length and complexity of the linguistic task is gradually increased from words to sentences.	SLP: **In this game, we're going to be working on talking slowly and smoothly. When it's our turn, we are going to say, "It's my turn now." Then we're going to say what color we got on the spinner such as "I got red." Remember to use your slow, smooth talking.** S: Spins and says **I got red** with slow, smooth speech.
7. Produces slow, smooth (easy) speech in structured tasks of gradually increasing complexity in the speech room in the presence of fluency disrupters, such as interruptions, contradictions, lack of eye contact, more people present, and so on.	SLP: **This morning your teacher read a story to your class. Did you like the story? Let's look at the pictures in the book she used and talk about them. As you talk, keep using your slow, smooth talking even if I interrupt you or don't seem to be listening to you.** S: Uses slow, smooth speech while talking about the story, even when there are disrupters.
Short-Term Goal: Transfers improved fluency to other environments and maintains it as it is achieved in each level	
8. Produces slow, smooth (easy) speech in spontaneous speech in phrases, sentences, and conversations with other people just outside the treatment setting.	SLP: **You're doing so well using your slow, smooth talking in our room. Now you're ready to start using your slow, easy speech outside our practice room. Your brother is going to meet us right outside our room in a few minutes. When you're talking to him, try to use your slow, easy speech while telling him about the game we played today.**

(continues)

Objectives	Examples
9. Produces slow, smooth (easy) speech in spontaneous speech in the presence of disrupters outside the treatment room (e.g., change the speaking setting, add interruptions and contradictions, have a lack of eye contact).	SLP: **At your house your parents have been your practice partners. This week when you're talking with your mom at home, keep using your slow, smooth talking even if she interrupts you or doesn't seem to be listening very well. Your mom is going to send me a note to let me know how you did.**
10. Maintains the use of slow, smooth (easy) speech and fluency as the frequency of formal speech treatment is gradually reduced.	SLP: **Using your slow, smooth talking seems to be a lot easier for you now. You're making great progress! Your parents and I have discussed how you will now be coming once a week instead of twice a week to speech.** S: Receives a good-progress certificate.

Older Students and Individuals With More Advanced Stuttering

Yearly Goal: *To communicate effectively in all speaking situations by using strategies that will enhance fluency and make stuttering easier*

Objectives	Examples
Short-Term Goal: Establishes the use of cognitive and self-instructional techniques that will facilitate the development of attitudes, self-concepts, and abilities that are consistent with long-term maintenance of improved fluency and an easier manner of stuttering	
1. Understands and applies knowledge of how speech is produced.	SLP: **Help me make a list of the parts of the body that are used for speaking as we look at this picture of a person's face and upper body. Later, we will talk about how they are used.** S: **lungs, vocal cords, diaphragm, jaw, teeth, tongue, lips, brain**
2. Discovers and describes the function of each body part used in speech production.	SLP: **You've named the parts of the body that make speech possible. Now let's see if we can figure out what each part does. What do you think the tongue does? What do the lungs do?** S: **The tongue helps you talk and eat; and the lungs help you talk and breathe.**
3. Demonstrates more knowledge about stuttering and how it differs from normal speech production.	SLP: **Today we're going to try to figure out how "normal" speech production is different from stuttered speech. Listen to these two ways of talking, and tell me how they are different: Can you see it? C-C-C-Caaan you see it?** S: **The first one was smooth and easy. The second one was bumpy. Your lips and neck were tense, and your tongue was pressing hard on the back of the roof of your mouth.**

Objectives	Examples
4. Demonstrates an understanding of what normal disfluencies are and what stuttering is by listing, describing, categorizing, and/or giving examples of each type. *Note: Normal disfluencies* include hesitation, interjection, revision, phrase repetition, and whole-word repetition. *Stuttered disfluencies* include whole-word repetition, part-word repetition, prolongation, block, and combinations of these.	SLP: **In our last session we talked about types of disfluencies. Today we're going to group them into normal disfluencies or stuttered disfluencies. I will write your answer in the normal disfluency column or the stuttered disfluency column. Listen to this one, and tell me what you hear: (1) I called Dave and asked him** (pause) **to come over. (2) Let mmmmmmmme sssssee. (3) My sister uh went to the um park. (4) Can you** (block) **see the board?** S: **(1) Normal disfluency, (2) stuttered disfluency, (3) normal disfluency, (4) stuttered disfluency.**
5. Identifies normal disfluencies and stuttered disfluencies in the speech of others and in his or her own speech.	SLP: **Today we're going to listen to a recording of some different speakers. Some will have normal disfluencies, and others will have stuttered disfluencies. Use the columns on this paper to make a tally mark in the column labeled *normal disfluency* or the one labeled *stuttered disfluency*. Let's do the first ones together: (1) And then—and then—the man came. (2) I w-w-w-want to buy iiice cream.** S: (1) Puts mark in normal disfluency column. (2) Puts mark in stuttered disfluency column.
6. Demonstrates understanding of the therapy process and the necessary commitment by consistently completing assignments and responding to questions.	SLP: **It's so important for both of us to be committed to working together. Lots of consistent work from both of us makes for success. I've noticed that you haven't done your homework from last week. Is there a reason? I know you wish the stuttering would just go away or get better on its own. I do, too, but we both know that's not how it works. Are your assignments too long? What can I do to help you?** S: Describes any difficulties and needs.
7. Identifies negative feelings and attitudes about speaking and stuttering and modifies them as necessary. *Teaching Note:* After the drawing is complete, discuss the drawing with regard to things in the picture that could represent negative feelings or feelings of being out of control, such as monsters, chains, and so on.	SLP: **Let's talk about how you feel about speaking and stuttering. Sometimes drawing can help us understand how we feel about things. I want you to draw a picture of your stuttering. Tell me how it makes you feel.** S: Draws picture and discusses feelings with the SLP.

(continues)

Objectives	Examples
8. Identifies positive personal qualities.	SLP: **Sometimes we don't notice the good things about our personalities. It's important to appreciate our good qualities. Trace your hand. On each finger, write something positive about yourself.** S: Writes words such as *good friend, thoughtful, kind,* and so on.
9. Lists situations in which she wants to develop use of improved fluency and easier stuttering, then arranges these in a hierarchical manner from easiest to hardest.	SLP: **Think of all of the social situations that you want to improve your speech in, and list them from easiest to hardest.** S: **(1) Talking to my best friend. (2) Talking to a friend while walking. (3) Answering a question in class.**
10. Describes and discusses stuttering openly and objectively with others and explains why it is important to be open.	SLP: **I'm sure that sometimes your friends or other people might call attention to or ask about your stuttering. What are some things you could say to them?** S: **Yeah, I stutter; it's no big deal. I'm working on it.**
11. Modifies stuttering to an easier form by stuttering openly without trying to hide it. *Note:* Over a period of time, the student begins to stutter more openly with the SLP and others, indicating increased acceptance of stuttering.	SLP: **What do I mean when I say "stutter openly"?** S: **Just let the stutter come out without trying to hide it.** SLP: **What are the consequences of trying to hide stuttering?** S: **It makes it even more difficult to talk fluently. I also miss out on a lot of times when I really wanted to say something.**
12. Identifies word and situation avoidance behaviors. *Note:* Word avoidance and situation avoidance are targeted separately.	SLP: **This week, I want you to make a list of some times you decide not to talk because you are afraid you will stutter. Put tally marks by situations that happen more than once. We will talk about your list next week.** S: Writes situations such as answering the phone and giving a report in class.
13. Decreases word and situation avoidances by being open about stuttering and using voluntary stuttering, positive self-talk, and other cognitive strategies.	SLP: **We are going to focus on one of the situations you listed last week where you avoided talking because of a fear of stuttering. Let's role-play your part in the group presentation and practice it until you are comfortable with your speech. Before we start, let's talk about what you will tell yourself to speak more fluently and use your easier stuttering.** S: **I will use easy onsets to increase fluency and pullouts to correct stuttering. I know my topic, which makes me confident about what I'm going to say.**

Objectives	Examples
14. Resists time pressures by delaying responses.	SLP: **What are some strategies you can use when you feel rushed to talk?** S: **When the teacher asks me a question in the classroom, I can count to 2 seconds before I answer. When the phone rings, I will count to 5 seconds before answering.**
15. Demonstrates a sense of being in control of his own speech by choosing which controls to use and when to use them.	SLP: **Because you told me that you will be doing an oral presentation in your class next week, let's talk about which controls you will use. Then we will practice them.** S: **I think I will choose to use slower speech and easy onsets to increase fluency when I stutter. I will use either cancellations or pullouts as corrections.**
Short-Term Goal: Improves overall communication abilities by developing an easier manner of stuttering consisting primarily of whole-word repetitions, easy one- to two-unit part-word repetitions, and easy prolongations	
16. Monitors the sensations associated with stuttering, giving specific descriptions of locations and degree of tension, and becomes desensitized to stuttering.	SLP: **Today we are going to be working on describing how stuttering feels. First, I'll stutter very hard with full tension, and then I want you to do it just like I did. Then I'll stutter with about half the tension, and I want you to do that one just like I did. (1) b-b-b-b-boat, (2) b-b-b-b-boat. What did you feel? Where was the tension? What is the difference between the first and second examples?** S: **On the first one, my lips pressed together with a lot of force, and on the second one, they touched together lightly. The second one had less tension and was easier.**

(continues)

Objectives	Examples
17. Identifies, analyzes, and models hard stuttering, easy stuttering, and fluent speech.	SLP: **The word *fluency* is all about the way one word flows into another. A *disfluency* is a break in the flow of speech. Today we'll describe the differences in the way each production feels to us. I'm going to say some sentences, and I want you to imitate how I said each one as closely as you can. Then I want you to tell me what you felt and the type of disfluency that was in the sentence. (1) Can you** (silent block) **see the meadow?** S: (1) Imitates first example. **I felt tension in my throat and stomach. I was completely blocked. No sound was coming out.** SLP: **(2) W-w-w-would you please read this part?** S: (2) Imitates second example. **I felt lots of tension in my neck and chest. During the part-word repetition, there were struggle sounds.** SLP: **(3) I'm going, I'm going, to the play.** S: (3) Imitates third example. **There was no excess tension. It was a phrase repetition.**
18. Modifies stuttering to an easier form by reducing pressure in the articulators and using slow, easy stuttering.	SLP: **While we're talking, try to use your slow, easy stuttering when you stutter. Then we'll stop and talk about how it felt different from your hard stuttering.** S: **My lips didn't feel tight. I wasn't pressing so hard. My jaw and even my shoulders felt relaxed when I stuttered.**
19. Modifies stuttering to an easier form by using cancellations, pullouts or stretched speech, and preparatory sets.	SLP: **Let's work on using pullouts to make stuttering easier. Remember, to do a pullout, you need to stay in the stuttering moment long enough to feel where the tension is and gradually release it. I'll say some sentences and use pullouts, and you say them after me: "I D-d-d-don't want to go to bed." What did you feel as you did the pullout?** S: **I felt less tension and easier speech with the pullout.**
Short-Term Goal: Improves overall communication abilities by developing a more fluent manner of speaking	
20. Releases excessive muscular tension in specific areas by imitating and performing exercises for relaxation.	SLP: **Today we are going to work on relaxing our muscles. I will go first. Do what I do.** SLP raises hands high into the air, stretching her body out. Then leans far over to one side and stretches and then does the same on the other side. **Now it's your turn.** S: Follows the leader and then becomes the leader.

Objectives	Examples
21. Releases excessive muscular tension in the upper body and vocal tract during speaking tasks of gradually increasing complexity.	SLP: **It is important for the speech muscles to be free of excessive tension when you are speaking. I want you to say each word on this list, and tell me if you felt any excessive tension in your upper body or speech muscles.** S: Reads each word and reports on the amount of tension in the upper body and speech muscles.
22. Develops appropriate respiratory coordination for speaking and uses this coordination consistently when speaking in situations of gradually increasing complexity.	SLP: **Today we'll work some more on breath support. While we're talking I want you to place your hand on your abdomen and feel how it moves in and out when you talk. As you breathe out, let a word glide gently on your breath and say these words after me. Say *hi*. Say *happy*. Say *honey*. Say *honeybees*. Say *happy honeybees*. Say *How are you?***
23. Uses appropriate phrasing strategies to assist in adequate breath control. *Note:* (1) A reading passage that the SLP has marked for places to pause. (2) A reading passage marked by the student. (3) A reading passage that is not marked. (4) Conversation.	SLP: **While we're talking I want you to break your sentences into phrases. This will help you maintain a slower rate and breath support. I'll give an example, and then you will do it: The bus / came early today. / We had to run / to catch it.**
24. Decreases rate of speaking.	SLP: **While we work on describing pictures, try to remember to pause after each phrase and lengthen the first vowel in the phrase.** S: **Mmyy horse / iiis in the field / wiiith her colt.**
25. Develops a more fluent manner of speaking and reading aloud by using a chosen fluency-shaping approach (e.g., prolonged speech such as the *easy relaxed approach: smooth movement* [ERA-SM] or *easy speaking voice* [ESV]) in tasks of gradually increasing complexity, both linguistically and socially.	SLP: **When you tell the class about your picture, remember to start with an easy onset or light contact. Make the first vowel slightly longer and return to a normal rate. You will need to do these things many times while you are telling the students about your picture.** S: Uses easy onset to say, **I drew this picture of my dog.**
26. Increases flexibility of speech by learning to vary rate, loudness, pause time, and so on.	SLP: **When you do your part in the group presentation next week, it will be more interesting if you change the rate, loudness, and pause time in your speech. Let's look at what you are going to say, and then mark some places where you could speak softer or louder, speak slower or more quickly, or make a pause.** S: Helps decide how to vary his speech, and then practices it with the SLP before presenting it to the class.

(continues)

Objectives	Examples
27. Understands and uses the communication skills of eye contact, phrasing, listening, and turn taking.	SLP: **There are some special skills that anyone can use to become a better communicator. Write down these words and then think of a picture you could draw to remind you to use these skills. They are eye contact, phrasing, listening, and turn taking.** S: **I will tell about turn taking. I can draw a picture of two people tossing a ball back and forth to remind me to take turns during a conversation.**

Maintenance and Transfer of Improved Fluency

Yearly Goal: *To transfer improved fluency and an easier manner of stuttering to other environments and maintain them*

Objectives	Examples
Short-Term Goal: Transfers improved fluency and an easier manner of stuttering to other environments	
1. Participates in a transfer program through all stages of treatment that will facilitate the use of the cognitive and self-instructional techniques, improved fluency, and easier manner of stuttering achieved in the therapy setting in other environments.	SLP: **Tomorrow you are going to a birthday party. Let's talk about what strategies you could use to help with smooth speech. We will practice telling your friend "happy birthday." What strategies will you use?** S: **I will use relaxed breath and easy onset when I tell Adam "happy birthday," like this: After I breathe in a relaxed way, I'll use an easy onset on the /h/ and say "hhhhappy birthday."**
Short-Term Goal: Maintains improved fluency and an easier manner of stuttering	
2. Maintains the use of improved fluency as the frequency of formal intervention is decreased.	SLP: **Because I don't see you as often anymore, I want to hear about how your speech has been. What are some ways you're using the techniques that you have found helpful?** S: **I've been using the light contact technique when I answer questions in class. For *pirate*, I touch my lips lightly together, and then move into my easy voice to finish the word.**
3. Uses information and strategies learned in therapy to problem solve and independently handle any relapses that occur after dismissal from formal speech treatment.	SLP: **When you notice more stuttering, what are you doing to help yourself?** S: **It reminds me that I may not be practicing as much as I should, so I will look in my notebook at the plan we made. That helps me get back into daily practice and reminds me of the strategies that work for me. I will remind myself to use my pullouts when I'm stuck.**

Objectives	Examples
4. If unable to handle relapses (see Objective 3), pursues formal "refresher" treatment as soon as the inability to regain control is realized.	SLP: **I'm glad you called me for a refresher time together. It was a smart thing to do. Let's talk about strategies to help you regain control.** S: **I need to talk about how to handle fluency disrupters like time pressures. I need to work on being more aware of easy breathing when I feel rushed.**

References

Introduction

American Speech-Language-Hearing Association. (n.d.). *Common Core State Standards: A resource for SLPs*. Retrieved December 21, 2014, from http://www.asha.org/SLP/schools/Common-Core-State Standards/

Barton, J., Lanza, J., & Wilson, C. (1983). *SCOR: Sequentional communication objectives for remediation*. Moline, IL: LinguiSystems.

Common Core State Standards Initiative. (2010). *Preparing America's students for college and career.* Retrieved from www.corestandards.org

Education for All Handicapped Children Act of 1975, 20 U.S.C. § 1400 *et seq.* (1975).

Hodge, M., & Wellma, L. (1999). Management of children with dysarthria. In A. Caruso & E. Strand (Eds.), *Clinical management of motor speech disorders in children*. New York, NY: Thieme.

Individuals With Disabilities Education Act of 1990, 20 U.S.C. § 1400 *et seq.* (1990) (amended 1997).

Kleim, J., & Jones, T. (2008). Principles of experience-dependent neural plasticity: Implications for rehabilitation after brain damage. *Journal of Speech, Language, and Hearing Research*, *51*, S225–S239.

Lass, N., & Pannbacker, M. (2008). The application of evidence-based practice to nonspeech oral motor treatment. *Language, Speech, and Hearing Services in the Schools*, *39*, 408–421.

Lof, G. (2008). Introduction to controversies about the use of nonspeech oral motor exercises. *Seminars in Speech and Language*, *29*(4), 253–256.

Lof, G. (2015, October 21). *Why nonspeech oral motor exercises (NSOME) do not work*. Presentation to Texas Christian University, Fort Worth, TX.

McCauley, R., Strand, E., Lof, G. L., Schooling, T., & Frymark, T. (2009). Evidence-based systematic review: Effects of nonspeech oral motor exercises on speech. *American Journal of Speech–Language Pathology*, *18*, 343–360.

Power-deFur, L. (2016). *Common Core State Standards and the speech–language pathologist: Standards-based intervention for special populations*. San Diego, CA: Plural.

Ruscello, D. (2008). Oral motor treatment issues related to children with developmental speech sound disorders. *Language, Speech, and Hearing Services in the Schools*, *39*, 380–391.

Subery, A., Wilson, E., Braddus, T., & Potter, N. (2006, November). *Tongue strength in preschool children: Measures, implications, and revelations*. Poster presented at the annual meeting of the American Speech-Language-Hearing Association, Miami Beach, FL.

Wightman, D., & Lintern, G. (1985). Part-task training of tracking manual control. *Human Factors*, *27*, 267–283.

Wilson, C., Lanza, J., & Evans, J. (1992). *The IEP companion: Communication goals for therapy in and out of the classroom*. East Moline, IL: LinguiSystems.

Wilson, E., Green, J., Yunusova, Y., & Morroe, C. (2008). Task specificity in early oral motor development. *Seminars in Speech and Language*, *29*(4), 257–265.

Winner, M., & Crooke, P. (2016). Beyond skills: The worth of social competence. *The ASHA Leader*, *21*, 50–56.

Unit 1: Pragmatics

Appel, K., & Masterson, J. (1998). *Assessment and treatment of narrative skills: What's the story?* Rockville, MD: ASHA.

Bloom, L., & Lahey, M. (1978). *Language development and language disorders*. New York, NY: John Wiley & Sons.

Cartledge, G., & Milburn, J. (1986). *Teaching social skills to children: Innovative approaches* (2nd ed.). New York, NY: Pergamon Press.

Chapman, R. (1981). Exploring children's communicative intents. In J. Miller (Ed.), *Assessing language production in children: Experimental procedures* (pp. 347–383). Austin, TX: PRO-ED.

Chomsky, N. (1999). On the nature, use, and acquisition of language. In W. Ritchie & T. Bhatia (Eds.), *Handbook of child language acquisition*. San Diego, CA: Academic Press.

Coggins, T., & Carpenter, R. (1981). The communicative intention inventory: A system for observing and coding children's early intentional communication. *Applied Psycholinguistics, 2*, 235–251.

Diamond, M., & Hopson, J. (1998). *Magic trees of the mind: How to nurture your child's intelligence, creativity, and healthy emotions from birth through adolescence*. New York, NY: Penguin Putnam.

Diamond, S. (2011). *Social rules for children: The top 100 social rules kids need to succeed*. Shawnee Mission, KS: AAPC.

Dore, J. (1975). Holophrases, speech acts, and language universals. *Journal of Child Language, 2*, 21–40.

Dore, J. (1978). Requestive systems in nursery school conversations: Analysis of talk in its social context. In R. Campbell & P. Smith (Eds.), *Recent advances in the psychology of language*. New York, NY: Plenum Press.

Duke, M., Nowicki, S., & Martin, E. (1996). *Teaching your child the language of social success*. Atlanta, GA: Peachtree.

Fey, M. (1986). *Language intervention with young children*. San Diego, CA: College-Hill Press.

Gleason, J., & Ratner, N. (2013). *The development of language* (8th ed.). Boston, MA: Pearson.

Gresham, F., & Elliott, S. (1990). *Social skills rating system: Manual*. Circle Pines, MN: American Guidance Service.

Gresham, F., & Elliott, S. (2008). *Social skills improvement system (SSIS) rating scales*. Circle Pines, MN: American Guidance Service.

Grice, H. (1975). Logic and conversation. In P. Cole & J. Morgan (Eds.), *Syntax and semantics*. New York, NY: Academic Press.

Halliday, M. A. (1975). *Learning how to mean: Explorations in the meaning of language*. New York, NY: Elsevier-North Holland.

Kowalski, T. (2002). *The source for Asperger's syndrome*. East Moline, IL: LinguiSystems.

Lanza, J., & Flahive, L. (2008). *Guide to communication milestones*. East Moline, IL: LinguiSystems.

Larson, V., & McKinley, N. (1995). *Language disorders in older students*. Eau Claire, WI: Thinking Publications.

Lindamood, P. C., & Lindamood, P. D. (2011). *LIPS: The Lindamood phoneme sequencing program for reading, spelling, and speech: Manual* (4th ed.). Austin, TX: PRO-ED.

Miller, J. (1981). *Assessing language production in children: Experimental procedures*. Austin, TX: PRO-ED.

Naremore, R., Densmore, A., & Harman, D. (2001). *Assessment and treatment of school-age language disorders: A resource manual*. San Diego, CA: Singular.

Ninio, A., & Snow, C. (1999). The development of pragmatics: Learning to use language appropriately. In W. Ritchie & T. Bhatia (Eds.), *Handbook of child language acquisition*. San Diego, CA: Academic Press.

Owens, R. (2016). *Language development: An introduction* (9th ed.). Boston, MA: Pearson.

Power-deFur, L. (2016). *Common Core State Standards and the speech–language pathologist: Standards-based intervention for special populations*. San Diego, CA: Plural.

Richard, G. (2000). *The source for treatment methodologies in autism*. East Moline, IL: LinguiSystems.

Strong, C. (1998). *The Strong narrative assessment procedure*. Eau Claire, WI: Thinking Publications.

Wiig, E., & Wilson, C. (2001). *Map it out: Visual tools for thinking, organizing, and communicating*. Eau Claire, WI: Thinking Publications.

Wilson, C. (1993). *Room 14: A social language program*. East Moline, IL: LinguiSystems.

Winner, M., & Crooke, P. (2016). Beyond skills: The worth of social competence. *The ASHA Leader, 21*, 50–56.

Unit 2: Vocabulary and Meaning

Beck, I., McKeown, M., & Kucan, L. (2003). *Bringing words to life: Robust vocabulary instruction*. New York, NY: Guilford Press.

Brown, B., & Edwards, M. (1989). *Developmental disorders of language*. London, UK: Whur.

Diamond, M., & Hopson, J. (1998). *Magic trees of the mind: How to nurture your child's intelligence, creativity, and healthy emotions from birth through adolescence*. New York, NY: Penguin Putnam.

Flahive, L., & Lanza, J. (2001). *Just for kids: Answering questions*. East Moline, IL: LinguiSystems.

Lanza, J., & Flahive, L. (2008). *Guide to communication milestones*. East Moline, IL: LinguiSystems.

Owens, R. (2010). *Language disorders: A functional approach to assessment and intervention* (5th ed.). Boston, MA: Allyn & Bacon.

Owens, R. (2014). *Language disorders: A functional approach to assessment and intervention* (6th ed.). New York, NY: Allyn & Bacon.

Schuele, C. M. (2011). *Vocabulary development in preschool children: ASHA language and literacy in preschool children.* ASHA online conference. Retrieved from www.asha.org

Wiig, E., & Semel, E. (1984). *Language assessment and intervention for the learning disabled* (2nd ed.). Columbus, OH: Charles E. Merrill.

Wiig, E., & Wilson, C. (2001). *Map it out: Visual tools for thinking, organizing, and communicating.* Eau Claire, WI: Thinking Publications.

Unit 3: Syntax and Morphology

Gleason, J. G. (2001). *The development of language* (5th ed.). Needham Heights, MA: Allyn & Bacon.

Lanza, J., & Flahive, L. (2008). *Guide to communication milestones.* East Moline, IL: LinguiSystems.

Owens, R. (1999). *Language disorders: A functional approach to assessment and intervention* (3rd ed.). Needham Heights, MA: Allyn & Bacon.

Owens, R. (2010). *Language disorders: A functional approach to assessment and intervention* (5th ed.). Boston, MA: Allyn & Bacon.

Owens, R. (2016). *Language development: An introduction* (9th ed.). Boston, MA: Pearson.

Wiig, E., & Semel, E. (1984). *Language assessment and intervention for the learning disabled* (2nd ed.). Columbus, OH: Charles E. Merrill.

Wilson, C., & Johnston, V. (1998). *SPARC for questions.* East Moline, IL: LinguiSystems.

Unit 4: Critical Thinking for Language and Communication

Bloom, B. (Ed.). (1956). *Taxonomy of educational objectives: The classification of educational goals. Handbook I: Cognitive domain.* New York, NY: David McKay.

Buttrill, J., Niizawa, J., Biemer, C., Takahashi, C., & Hearn, S. (1989). Serving the language learning disabled adolescent: A strategies-based model. *Language, Speech, and Hearing Services in Schools, 20,* 185–204.

Costa, A., & Lowery, L. (1989). *Techniques for teaching thinking.* Pacific Grove, CA: Midwest Publications.

De Bono, E. (1994). *De Bono's thinking course* (Rev. ed.). New York, NY: Facts on File.

Gardner, H. (1983). *Frames of mind: The theory of multiple intelligences.* New York, NY: Basic Books.

Jones, C. (2002). *The source for brain-based learning.* East Moline, IL: LinguiSystems.

Kowalski, T. (2002). *The source for Asperger's syndrome.* East Moline, IL: LinguiSystems.

Letuchy, S. (2015). *The visual edge: Graphic organizers for standards based learning.* Indianapolis, IN: Dog Ear.

Lujan, M. (2003). *Critical thinking reference.* Tyler, TX: Teacher Resources.

Nelson, N. (2010). *Language and literacy disorders: Infancy through adolescence.* Boston, MA: Allyn & Bacon.

Owens, R. (2010). *Language disorders: A functional approach to assessment and intervention* (5th ed.). Boston, MA: Allyn & Bacon.

Richards, R. (1999). *The source for learning and memory strategies.* East Moline, IL: LinguiSystems.

Wiig, E., Larson, V., & Olson, J. (2004). *S-maps: Rubrics for curriculum-based assessment and intervention.* Eau Claire, WI: Thinking Publications.

Wiig, E., & Semel, E. (1984). *Language assessment and intervention for the learning disabled* (2nd ed.). Columbus, OH: Charles E. Merrill.

Wiig, E., & Wilson, C. (1994). Is a question a question? Passage understanding by preadolescents with learning disability. *Language, Speech, and Hearing Services in Schools, 25,* 241–250.

Wiig, E., & Wilson, C. (2001). *Map it out: Visual tools for thinking, organizing, and communicating.* Eau Claire, WI: Thinking Publications.

Winner, M., & Crooke, P. (2016). Beyond skills: The worth of social competence. *The ASHA Leader, 21,* 50–56.

Unit 5: Organization and Study Skills

Keeley, S. (2003). *The source for executive function disorders*. East Moline, IL: LinguiSystems.

Kowalski, T. (2002). *The source for Asperger's syndrome*. East Moline, IL: LinguiSystems.

Larson, V., & McKinley, N. (1995). *Language disorders in older students*. Eau Claire, WI: Thinking Publications.

Nelson, N. (2010). *Language and literacy disorders: Infancy through adolescence*. Boston, MA: Allyn & Bacon.

Robinson, A. (1993). *What smart students know*. New York, NY: Random House.

Wiig, E., Larson, V., & Olson, J. (2004). *S-maps: Rubrics for curriculum-based assessment and intervention*. Eau Claire, WI: Thinking Publications.

Unit 6: Listening

American Speech-Language-Hearing Association. (2005). *(Central) auditory processing disorders [Technical Report]*. Retrieved from www.asha.org

Bellis, T. J. (2004). Redefining auditory processing disorder: An audiologist's perspective. *The ASHA Leader, 9*(7), 7–22.

Graser, N. S. (1992). *125 ways to be a better listener*. East Moline, IL: LinguiSystems.

Justice, L. (2010). *Communication sciences and disorders: A contemporary perspective* (2nd ed.). Boston, MA: Allyn & Bacon.

Lindamood, P. C., & Lindamood, P. D. (2011). *LIPS: The Lindamood phoneme sequencing program for reading, spelling, and speech: Manual* (4th ed.). Austin, TX: PRO-ED.

Moore, B., & Montgomery, J. (2008). *Making a difference for America's children: Speech–language pathologists in public schools*. Greenville, SC: Thinking Publications.

Myklebust, H. R. (1954). *Auditory disorders in children: A manual for differential diagnosis*. New York, NY: Grune & Stratton.

Richard, G. (2001). *The source for processing disorders*. East Moline, IL: LinguiSystems.

Richard, G. (2004). Redefining auditory processing disorder: A speech–language pathologist's perspective. *The ASHA Leader, 9*(7), 7–22.

Winner, M., & Crooke, P. (2016, September). Beyond skills: The worth of social competence. *The ASHA Leader, 21*, 50–56.

Unit 7: Literacy: Reading

Calkins, L. (2001). *The art of teaching reading*. New York, NY: Longman.

Common Core State Standards Initiative. (2010). *Preparing America's students for college and career*. Retrieved from www.corestandards.org

Crow, L., & Reichmuth, S. (2001). *The source for early literacy development*. East Moline, IL: LinguiSystems.

Flahive, L., & Lanza, J. (2004). *Phonological awareness cards*. East Moline, IL: LinguiSystems.

Gillon, G. (2004). *Phonological awareness: From research to practice*. New York, NY: Guilford Press.

Hyerle, D. (1996). *Visual tools for constructing knowledge*. Alexandria, VA: Association for Supervision and Curriculum Development.

Inspiration (9th ed.) [Computer software]. (2016). Portland, OR: Inspiration Software.

Justice, L. (2010). *Communication sciences and disorders: A contemporary perspective* (2nd ed.). Boston, MA: Allyn & Bacon.

Lanza, J., & Flahive, L. (2008). *Guide to communication milestones*. East Moline, IL: LinguiSystems.

Letuchy, S. (2015). *The visual edge: Graphic organizers for standards based learning*. Indianapolis, IN: Dog Ear.

Lindamood, P. C., & Lindamood, P. D. (2011). *LIPS: The Lindamood phoneme sequencing program for reading, spelling, and speech: Manual* (4th ed.). Austin, TX: PRO-ED.

Owens, R. (2014). *Language disorders: A functional approach to assessment and intervention* (6th ed.). New York, NY: Allyn & Bacon.

Owens, R. (2016). *Language development: An introduction* (9th ed.). Boston, MA: Pearson.

Richards, R. (1999). *The source for dyslexia and dysgraphia*. East Moline, IL: LinguiSystems.

Robertson, S. (2002). *Read with me: Stress-free strategies for building language and listening*. Eau Claire, WI: Thinking Publications.

Robinson, A. (1993). *What smart students know.* New York, NY: Random House.

Shaywitz, S. (2005). *Overcoming dyslexia: A new and complete science-based program for reading problems at any level.* New York, NY: Alfred A. Knopf.

Snow, C., Scarborough, H., & Burns, M. (1999). What speech–language pathologists need to know about early reading. *Topics in Language Disorders, 20*(1), 48–58.

Stockdale, C., & Possin, C. (2001). *The source for solving reading problems.* East Moline, IL: LinguiSystems.

Swigert, N. (2004). *The source for reading fluency.* Austin, TX: PRO-ED.

Wiig, E., & Wilson, C. (2001). *Map it out: Visual tools for thinking, organizing, and communicating.* Eau Claire, WI: Thinking Publications.

Wiig, E., & Wilson, C. (2002). *The learning ladder: Assessing and teaching text comprehension.* Eau Claire, WI: Thinking Publications.

Unit 8: Literacy: Writing

American Speech-Language-Hearing Association. (2001). *Roles and responsibilities of speech–language pathologists with respect to reading and writing in children and adolescents* (guidelines) (ASHA Supplement 21, pp. 17–27). Rockville, MD: Ad Hoc Committee on Reading and Written Language Disorders.

Gleason, J., & Ratner, N. (2013). *The development of language* (8th ed.). Boston, MA: Pearson.

Graham, S., & Harris, K. (1999). Assessment and intervention in overcoming writing difficulties: An illustration from the self-regulation strategy development model. *Language, Speech, and Hearing Services in Schools, 30*, 255–264.

Inspiration (9th ed.) [Computer software]. (2016). Portland, OR: Inspiration Software.

Larson, V., & McKinley, N. (1995). *Language disorders in older students.* Eau Claire, WI: Thinking Publications.

Letuchy, S. (2015). *The visual edge: Graphic organizers for standards based learning.* Indianapolis, IN: Dog Ear.

Owens, R. (2010). *Language disorders: A functional approach to assessment and intervention* (5th ed.). Boston, MA: Allyn & Bacon.

Owens, R. (2014). *Language disorders: A functional approach to assessment and intervention* (6th ed.). New York, NY: Allyn & Bacon.

Richard, G. (2001). *The source for processing disorders.* East Moline, IL: LinguiSystems.

Richards, R. (1999). *The source for dyslexia and dysgraphia.* East Moline, IL: LinguiSystems.

Robinson, A. (1993). *What smart students know.* New York, NY: Random House.

Shaywitz, S. (2003). *Overcoming dyslexia: A new and complete science-based program for reading problems at any level.* New York, NY: Alfred A. Knopf.

Wiig, E., Larson, V., & Olson, J. (2004). *S-maps: Rubrics for curriculum-based assessment and intervention.* Eau Claire, WI: Thinking Publications.

Wiig, E., & Wilson, C. (1994). Is a question a question? Passage understanding by preadolescents with learning disability. *Language Speech, and Hearing Services in Schools, 25*(4), 241–250.

Unit 9: Speech Production

Bernthal, J., Bankson, N., & Flipsen, P. (Eds.). (2013). *Articulation and phonological disorders: Speech sound disorders in children* (7th ed.). Needham Heights, MA: Allyn & Bacon.

Bishop, D., & Adams, C. (1990). A prospective study of the relationship between specific language impairment, phonological disorders and reading retardation. *Journal of Child Psychology and Psychiatry, 31*(7), 1027–1050.

Creaghead, N., Newman, P., & Secord, W. (1989). *Assessment and remediation of articulatory and phonological disorders.* Columbus, OH: Merrill.

Flahive, L., & Lanza, J. (1998). *Just for kids: Phonological processing.* East Moline, IL. LinguiSystems.

Hegde, M. (1985). *Treatment procedures in communicative disorders.* Boston, MA: College-Hill Press.

Hodson, B. (2011). Enhancing phonological patterns of young children with highly unintelligible speech. *The ASHA Leader, 16*, 16–19.

Hodson, B., & Paden, E. (1991). *Targeting intelligible speech: A phonological approach to remediation* (2nd ed.). Austin, TX: PRO-ED.

Kent, R. (1998). Normal aspects of articulation. In J. Bernthal & N. Bankson (Eds.), *Articulation and phonological disorders* (4th ed.). Needham Heights, MA: Allyn & Bacon.

Lanza, J., & Flahive, L. (2008). *Guide to communication milestones*. East Moline, IL: LinguiSystems.

Mullen, R., & Schooling, T. (2010). The national outcomes measurement system for speech–language pathology. *Language, Speech, and Hearing Services in Schools, 41*, 44–60.

Peña-Brooks, A., & Hegde, M. (2000). *Assessment and treatment of articulation and phonological disorders in children*. Austin, TX: PRO-ED.

Weiss, C., Gordon, M., & Lillywhite, H. (1987). *Articulatory and phonologic disorders*. Baltimore, MD: Williams & Wilkins.

Unit 10: Voice

Boone, D. (2015). *Is your voice telling on you? How to find and use your natural voice* (3rd ed.). San Diego, CA: Plural.

Boone, D., McFarlane, S., Von Berg, S., & Zraick, R. (2010). *The voice and voice therapy* (8th ed.). New York, NY: Allyn & Bacon.

Chamberlain, C., & Strode, R. (1992). *Easy does it for voice*. East Moline, IL: LinguiSystems.

Greene, M. C., & Mathieson, L. (1992). *The voice and its disorders* (5th ed.). San Diego, CA: Singular.

Justice, L. (2010). *Communication sciences and disorders: A contemporary perspective* (2nd ed.). Boston, MA: Allyn & Bacon.

Stern, D. A. (2006). *The sound and style of American English* (3rd ed.) [Audio CD]. Lyndonville, VT: Dialect Accent Specialists.

Unit 11: Fluency

Adraensens, S., & Struyf, E. (2016). Secondary school teachers' beliefs, attitudes, and reactions to stuttering. *Language, Speech, and Hearing Services in Schools, 47*, 135–147.

Allen, M. (2007a). *Speak freely: Essential speech skills for school-age children who stutter* (Student workbook). Evanston, IL: Speak Freely Publications.

Allen, M. (2007b). *Speak freely: Essential speech skills for school-age children who stutter* (Therapist handbook). Evanston, IL: Speak Freely Publications.

Chmela, K., & Reardon, N. (2001). *The school-age child who stutters: Working effectively with attitudes and emotions; A workbook* (L. S. Trautman, Ed.). Memphis, TN: Stuttering Foundation of America.

Chmela, K., & Reardon, N. (2006). *Focus on fluency: A tool kit for creative therapy*. Greenville, SC: Super Duper Publications.

Dahye, C., Conture, E. G., Walden, T. A., Jones, R. M., & Hanjoe, K. (2016). Emotional diathesis, emotional stress, and childhood stuttering. *Journal of Speech, Language, and Hearing Research, 59*, 616–630.

Davidow, J. H., Zaroogian, L., & Garcia-Barrera, M. A. (2016). Strategies for teachers to manage stuttering in the classroom: A call for research. *Language, Speech, and Hearing Services in Schools, 15*, 1–14.

Gregory, H. (2003). *Stuttering therapy: Rationale and procedures*. Boston, MA: Allyn & Bacon.

Heinze, B., & Johnson, K. (1998). *Easy does it for fluency: Intermediate 2*. Austin, TX: PRO-ED.

Johnston, V. (2016). *Ways to help children improve their fluency: Suggestions for parents*. Retrieved from www.overtonspeech.net

Manning, W. (2001). *Decision making in fluency disorders*. San Diego, CA: Singular Publishing Group.

Nippold, M. (2012). When a school-age child stutters, let's focus on the primary problem. *Language, Speech, and Hearing Services in Schools, 43*, 549–551.

Van Riper, C. (1971). *The nature of stuttering*. Englewood Cliffs, NJ: Prentice Hall.

Van Riper, C. (1973). *The treatment of stuttering*. Englewood Cliffs, NJ: Prentice Hall.

Walton, P., & Wallace, M. (1998). *Fun with fluency: Direct therapy with the young child*. Bisbee, AZ: Imaginart.

Yaruss, J. S., Coleman, C. E., & Quesal, R. W. (2012). Stuttering in school-age children: A comprehensive approach to treatment. *Language, Speech, and Hearing Services in Schools, 43*, 536–548.

Appendixes

Fokes, J. (1976). *Fokes sentence builder instructor's guide*. New York, NY: Teaching Resources.

Gess, D. (2006). *Teaching writing: Strategies for improving literacy across the curriculum* (2nd ed.). Suffern, NY: ERA/CCR Corporation, The Write Track.

Hyerle, D. (1996). *Visual tools for constructing knowledge*. Alexandria, VA: Association for Supervision and Curriculum Development.

Inspiration (9th ed.) [Computer software]. (2016). Portland, OR: Inspiration Software.

Johnston, V. (2004). *Ways to help children improve their fluency: Suggestions for parents*. Retrieved from www.overtonspeech.net

Nelson, N. (1988). *Planning individualized speech and language intervention programs*. Austin, TX: PRO-ED.

Owens, R. (2014). *Language disorders: A functional approach to assessment and intervention* (6th ed.). New York, NY: Allyn & Bacon.

Richards, R. (1999). *The source for dyslexia and dysgraphia*. East Moline, IL: LinguiSystems.

Robertson, S. (2002). *Read with me: Stress-free strategies for building language and listening*. Eau Claire, WI: Thinking Publications.

Wiig, E., & Wilson, C. (2001). *Map it out: Visual tools for thinking, organizing, and communicating*. Eau Claire, WI: Thinking Publications.

Wilkes, E. (1999). *Cottage acquisition scales for listening, language, and speech: Pre-sentence level*. San Antonio, TX: Sunshine Cottage School for Deaf Children.

General

Nicolosi, L., Harryman, E., & Kresheck, J. (1989). *Terminology of communication disorders: Speech–language–hearing*. Baltimore, MD: Williams & Wilkins.

Richard, G., & Hoge, D. (1999). *The source for syndromes*. East Moline, IL: LinguiSystems.

Richard, G., & Hoge, D. (2000). *The source for syndromes 2*. East Moline, IL: LinguiSystems.

Appendix A

First Words

Receptive Words

9 months	16–18 months	22–24 months
Mommy	3 more foods	3 more body parts
10–12 months	5 more objects/activities	4 more commands
Daddy	4 animals	Words for:
no-no	1 command (no context clues)	indoors
bye	3 more names	outdoors
more	**19–21 months (100 total)**	community
up	3 more toys	vehicles
hot	4 more foods	buildings
bottle	4 more clothes	household
open	4 more animals	stores
all gone	2 more names	shopping
pet's name	15 more objects/activities	appliances
child's name	2 pronouns (*my, mine, me, you*)	tools
13–15 months (3–20 total)	3 adjectives	sports
3 toys	10 verbs	holidays
3 foods	2 or 3 songs	feelings
2 clothes	2 stories	values
4 objects/activities		attributes
2 body parts		Where?
		What's that?
		in
		on

Expressive Words

13–15 months (1 word), 16–18 months (10 words), 19–21 months (20+ words), 22–24 months (50–75 words)

Social words	Demanding words	Nouns
no-no	*up*	3 toys
sh!	*more*	3 foods
bye-bye	*off*	2 body parts
hi	*out*	2 clothes
uh-oh	*gimme*	2 animals and/or animal sounds
ow!	*down*	3 household items
night-night		2 outside objects

(continues)

Social words

mmm! (*yummy*)

one of any other social routine (e.g., *kisses, so big*)

Important people	**Telling words**	**Verbs**
Mama	*all gone*	*open*
Daddy	*here*	*eat*
child's name	*there*	*sleep*
pet's name	*dirty*	*look* (or *lookit*)
1 or 2 names of other people	*hot*	3 other verbs
	that	

Note: Adapted from *Cottage Acquisition Scales for Listening, Language, and Speech,* by E. Wilkes, 1999, San Antonio, TX: Sunshine Cottage School for Deaf Children.

Appendix B

Word Lists

Labels and Categories

Action labels	Body parts	Animals
drink	eyes	cat, kitty
eat	mouth	dog, puppy
cry	nose	cow
come	ears	duck
sleep	hair	pig
go	arms	bird
see	legs	bug
hug	stomach, tummy	goat
Food and drink	**Toys**	**Animal categories**
milk	ball	farm
cookie	doll	zoo
juice	car	jungle
water	book	woods
bread	swing	swimming
chips	tricycle	flying
apple	truck	rain forest
banana	bear	desert
Places (names)	**Furniture**	**General household**
bye-bye	bed	bathroom
home	chair	bedroom
store	table	closet
place of worship	couch, sofa	window
school	desk	ceiling
restaurants	dresser	floor
hospital	lamp	door
street		kitchen
park		
School	**Vehicles**	**Occupations**
classroom	car	teacher
teacher	truck	police officer
paper	airplane	firefighter
scissors	train	doctor
pencil	bus	nurse

(continues)

Labels and Categories

School	Vehicles	Occupations
crayons	boat	mail carrier
glue	bicycle	pilot
playground	SUV	dentist
		Shapes
		circle
		square
		triangle
		rectangle
		oval
		diamond

Position Concepts (Prepositions)

Ages at which position concepts emerge in most children (Nelson, 1988)

2-0 to 3-0	3-0 to 4-0	4-0 to 5-0	5-0 to 6-0
in	up	beside	behind
off	top	bottom	ahead of
on	around	backward	first
under	high	forward	last
out of	in front of	down	
together	in back of	low	
away from	next to	between	
		inside	
Additional concepts			
above–below	outside–inside	through	right–left
over–under	middle	near–far	after–before

Quality Concepts (Adjectives)

Size	Quantity	Attractiveness
big–little	more–less	ugly–pretty
large–small	all–none	nice
medium	empty–full	clean–dirty
enormous, huge–tiny	each	
	many–few	
	some–all	
Taste, smell	**Temperature**	**Colors**
sweet–sour	hot–cold	red
awful	chilly–warm	blue
fragrant	cool–warm	yellow

(continues)

Quality Concepts (Adjectives)

Taste, smell
delicious
good
bad
salty

Length, height, width
long–short
thin–fat
tall–short
wide–narrow
thick–thin
skinny–fat

Feelings
happy, glad
loved
proud
glad
calm
patient
hopeful
excited
surprised
sad
shy
embarrassed
tired
bored
sorry
guilty
jealous
angry, mad
hurt
scared, afraid

Sound
loud–quiet
noisy–quiet
roaring–silent
whirring
dripping
splashing
chiming

Other concepts
hot–cold
happy–sad
fast–slow
same–different
hard–soft
old–young
new–old
rough–smooth
wet–dry
strong–weak
light–heavy
crooked–straight
broken
funny
spotted
beautiful–ugly
curly–straight
dark–light
good–bad
mean
careful
sharp–dull
squishy
scratchy

Colors
green
orange
black
brown
purple
white
violet
tan
gray

Temporal Concepts

See Owens (2014).

next	today	days
before	tomorrow	weeks
after	calendar dates	hours
into	months	minutes
soon	seasons	through
later	numerals for years	away from
now	morning	toward
above	afternoon	sometimes
yesterday	evening	

Plurals

Regular		
-s	*-es*	Change *f* to *v*, add *-es*
ants	boxes	calves
apples	dishes	knives
balloons	glasses	leaves
cows	sandwiches	lives
doctors	watches	loaves
letters	foxes	wives
mechanics	dresses	wolves
shoes		
Irregular		
cattle	moose	
children	fish	
clothes	sheep	
deer	teeth	
men		

Pronouns

Personal pronouns	Possessive pronouns	Reflexive pronouns	Relative pronouns
I, me	my, mine	myself	this
you	your, yours	yourself	these
he, she, it	his, its	himself	that
him, her	her, hers	herself	those
they, them	they, theirs	itself	
we, us	our, ours	ourselves	
		yourselves	
		themselves	

(continues)

Pronouns

Indefinite pronouns		
all	everybody	no one
another	everyone	one
any	few	other
anybody	many	several
anyone	most	some
both	neither	somebody
each	nobody	someone
either	none	such

Irregular Past Tense Verbs

ate	dug	read	swung
bent	fed	rode	threw
blew	fell	sang	took
broke	flew	sat	tore
built	found	saw	was
came	gave	shut	went
caught	got	slept	were
cut	had	slid	won
did	held	spread	wore
dived, dove	hurt	stood	wrote
drank	lost	strung	
drew	put	swam	
drove	ran	swept	

Conjunctions

Listed in the order of acquisition. See Owens (2014).

and	because	although, while, as
and then	so, if, when	unless
but, or	until, before, after	therefore, however

Transition Words

To indicate a sequence (*then* relations)

first, at first
then, after that
next, still, too
finally, eventually
for example
also, furthermore
soon, as soon as
first, second, third

To indicate an example (descriptive relations)

in addition to
besides
for example
such as
for instance

To indicate time (temporal relations)

after a while
as soon as
before
at last
immediately
in the past
meanwhile
shortly
since
until
when

To compare or contrast (comparative relations)

although
however
in comparison
in contrast
likewise
nevertheless
on the other hand
similarly, whereas, yet

To indicate cause–effect (causal relations)

because, because of
due to
so, so that
therefore
in order to
thus
since
consequently
as a result
if–then

Summary, repetition, or conclusion

as a result
as I have said
as we have seen
as mentioned earlier
in any event
in conclusion
therefore
to summarize

Modal Auxiliaries

can	need to
could	ought to
have to	shall
may	should
might	will
must	would

Antonyms

Level I	Level II
asleep–awake	crooked–straight
big–little	deep–shallow
black–white	fast–slow
boy–girl	first–last
closed–open	lock–unlock
cold–hot	lose–find
come–go	loud–quiet
day–night	loud–soft
empty–full	many–few
fat–skinny	near–far
front–back	old–young
high–low	rich–poor
in–out	rough–smooth
left–right	same–different
long–short	sharp–dull
mother–father	sick–well
old–new	south–north
on–off	summer–winter
pull–push	sweet–sour
run–walk	tall–short
sad–happy	thick–thin
soft–hard	tight–loose
stand–sit	ugly–pretty
stop–go	wide–narrow
throw–catch	work–play
top–bottom	
under–over	
up–down	
wet–dry	
yes–no	

Synonyms

Level I

hat–cap
coat–jacket
rug–carpet
street–road
icebox–refrigerator
glue–paste
pants–slacks–trousers–jeans
freeway–highway
store–shop
well–healthy
sick–ill
laugh–giggle–chuckle
mad–angry–furious
night–evening
girl–female
boy–male
fast–quick–speedy–swift
happy–glad
car–automobile
over–above

Synonyms

Level II

baby–infant	bold–courageous	restaurant–cafe
sleep–slumber	couch–sofa–divan	old–ancient
billfold–wallet	funny–hilarious	ugly–unattractive
cook–chef	job–occupation–career	brag–boast
buy–purchase	teacher–instructor	want–desire
seldom–infrequent	walk–stroll	habitual–usual
empty–void		

Multiple-Meaning Words

batter	board	bridge	brook
buckle	carriage	choice	course
court	crop	cross	drag
ear	film	finish	float
gather	grain	graze	ground
harness	heart	idle	key
line	list	mean	mill
mind	note	part	pass
pepper	pick	point	pupil
rent	rest	round	shade
sharp	shed	shell	shock
short	slip	snug	square
stall	step	stick	suit
thread			

Homonyms

ate–eight	aunt–ant	base–bass	bear–bare	beet–beat
berry–bury	brake–break	dear–deer	eye–I	fair–fare
flower–flour	hair–hare	hear–here	hole–whole	hose–hoes
mail–male	meat–meet–mete	night–knight	pain–pane	pale–pail
pear–pair–pare	peek–peak	plane–plain	rain–rein	read–reed
right–write	root–route	sale–sail	sea–see	shoot–chute
so–sew	some–sum	son–sun	stair–stare	steak–stake
tail–tale	to–two–too	wait–weight	way–weigh	wood–would

Verbal Analogies

Whole–part

A leg is to a knee as an arm is to an elbow.

A school is to a classroom as a house is to a kitchen.

A tennis shoe is to a shoelace as a computer is to a keyboard.

A bird is to a beak as a bear is to a claw.

A pizza is to a slice as ice cream is to a scoop.

Part–whole

An orange is to a tree as a blackberry is to a bush.

A word is to a sentence as a letter is to a word.

A week is to a month as a chapter is to a book.

A sleeve is to a shirt as a branch is to a tree.

A musical note is to a song as a word is to a story.

Object–action

A bike is to riding as a racket is to hitting.

A pencil is to writing as a paintbrush is to painting.

A spoon is to stirring as a knife is to cutting.

A ladder is to climbing as a hammer is to hitting.

Yarn is to knitting as thread is to sewing.

Action–object

Ringing is to a bell as honking is to a horn.

Digging is to a shovel as raking is to a rake.

Eating is to a fork as drinking is to a straw.

Hearing is to an ear as seeing is to an eye.

Sitting is to a chair as sleeping is to a bed.

Location

A person is to a house as a bird is to a nest.

A hat is to a head as a shoe is to a foot.

A fish is to a lake as a bird is to the sky.

A flower is to a plant as an apple is to a tree.

A car is to a garage as a cow is to a barn.

Antonym

Up is to down as over is to under.

First is to last as most is to least.

Big is to little as tall is to short.

Sad is to happy as mean is to nice.

Hot is to cold as bumpy is to smooth.

Synonym

Happy is to cheerful as miserable is to sad.

A duet is to two as a trio is to three.

Whisper is to yell as laugh is to cry.

Intelligent is to smart and thoughtful is to kind.

Wealthy is to rich as bashful is to shy.

Time

A second is to a minute as a minute is to an hour.

A day is to a week as a week is to a month.

A season is to a year as a year is to a decade.

Thirty minutes is to an hour as six months is to a year.

A week is to a month as a month is to a year.

Familial

A mother is to a father as a sister is to a brother.

Aunt is to niece as uncle is to nephew.

Uncle is to he as aunt is to she.

Daughter is to mother as son is to father.

Rooster is to hen as husband is to wife.

Sequence reversal

May is to April as July is to June.

Finish is to start as dessert is to appetizer.

Second is to first as fourth is to third.

Morning is to dawn as night is to afternoon.

The letter G is to H as the letter P is to O.

Grammatical

Tall is to taller as short is to shorter.

Boy is to boys as child is to children.

Man is to men as woman is to women.

Look is to looked as shout is to shouted.

Mouse is to mice as goose is to geese.

Figurative Language

Common idioms	Common similes	Common metaphors
big shot	warm as toast	He's an old bear.
dress up	weak as a kitten	She's a jewel.
catch a cold	cold as ice	He's a clown.

Common proverbs

Don't count your chickens before they're hatched.

Don't put all your eggs in one basket.

A penny saved is a penny earned.

Appendix C

Practical Reading Comprehension Ideas: Visual Organizers

There are many ways that speech–language pathologists (SLPs) can provide significant support to students who struggle with reading as an aspect of their language disorders, learning disabilities, auditory processing disorders, or visual memory problems.

These supports are *pre-reading*, *echo reading*, *paired reading*, and *visual organizers*. For example, you can use books that a young child is reading in the classroom and *pre-read* the book with her using echo reading or paired reading (Robertson, 2002). In echo reading, the SLP reads a short phrase and then says to the child, "Copy me." Through use of echo reading with an adult, children will likely advance their emerging reading skills, and they will gain confidence in their ability to eventually read a book independently. Comprehension improves when children hear a story read fluently without first struggling to decode every word. In paired reading, the SLP reads a part of a sentence (or page), and then has the child take a turn reading the next part. Paired reading helps children improve comprehension, intonation, and stress. Books with predictable story parts help emerging readers read their part with confidence.

Some students learn to read aloud fluently yet need intervention because their comprehension lags behind. For many students—especially those with language disorders, learning disabilities, or both—concept maps, discussed next, can provide a means of understanding complex relationships that these students do not grasp when described only in words.

Using concept maps as *visual organizers* relieves the burden on a student's auditory processing and memory abilities. That is because visual organizers help structure thinking and bring the critical thinking process to a conscious level. Students can refer to concept maps while engaged in thinking, organizing, and discussing what they have read. The process of making their own maps allows students with visual memory problems to store the conceptual maps of their mental models, provided the maps are not too complex. Thus, students construct an internal model that then helps them anticipate the structure of both literary and informational text. The improved comprehension not only increases knowledge but also builds confidence that extends into the next reading experience (Wiig & Wilson, 2001).

The maps in this appendix are provided as examples. There are many resources for various types of visual organizers for reading, writing, and critical thinking. Among those are *Visual Tools for Constructing Knowledge* (Hyerle, 1996), *The Source for Dyslexia and Dysgraphia* (Richards, 1999), and *Map It Out: Visual Tools for Thinking, Organizing, and Communicating* (Wiig & Wilson, 2001). Students can also create their own concept maps. They can draw them or use computer programs. The user-friendly program *Inspiration 9.0* can be downloaded from the Internet. This resource allows students in Grades K–12 to create colorful concept maps and other visual organizers (Inspiration, 2016).

Visual Organizers

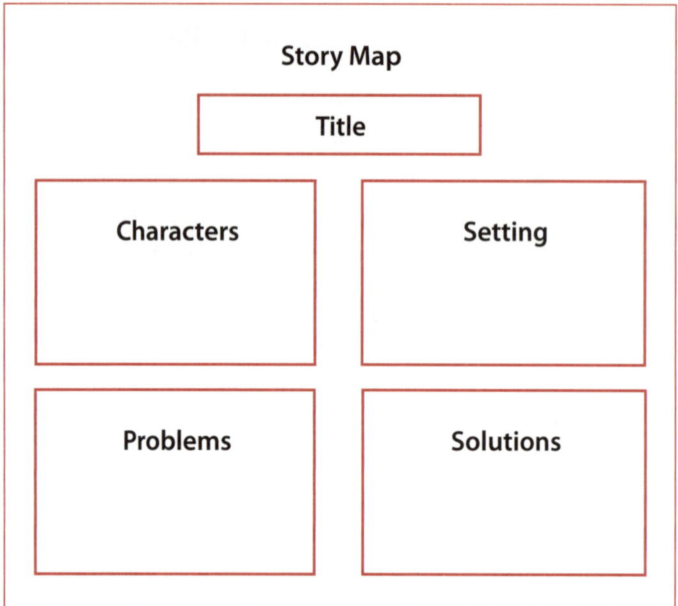

Figure C-1

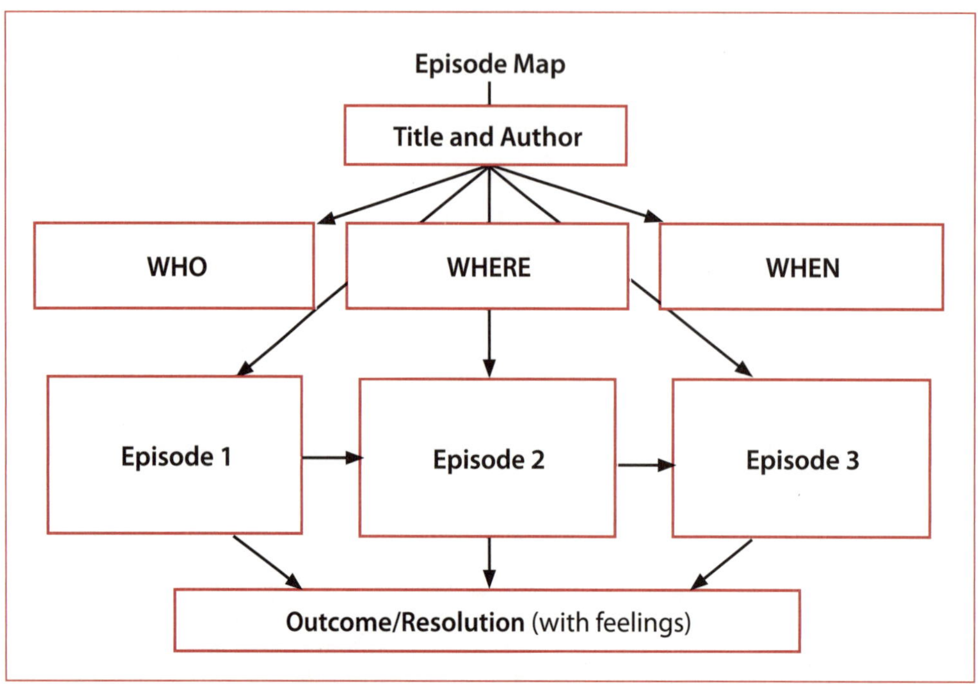

Figure C-2

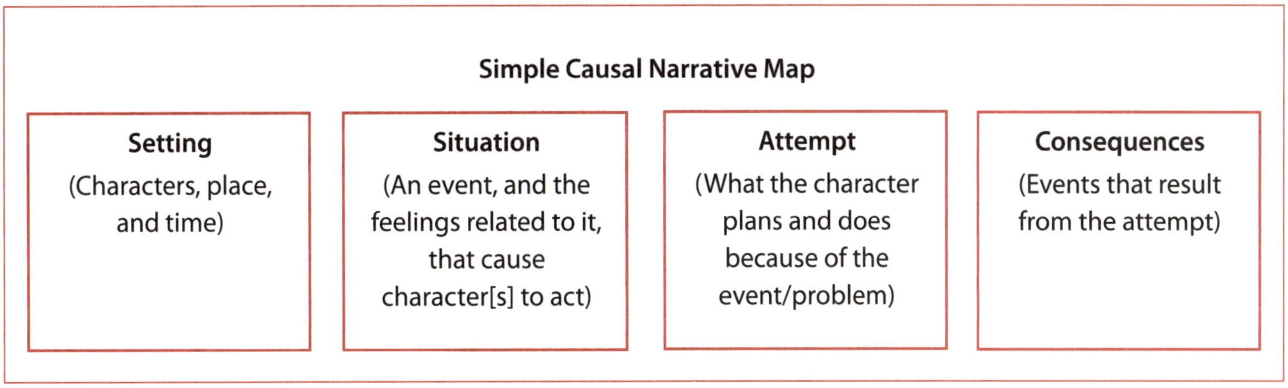

Simple Causal Narrative Map

Setting	Situation	Attempt	Consequences
(Characters, place, and time)	(An event, and the feelings related to it, that cause character[s] to act)	(What the character plans and does because of the event/problem)	(Events that result from the attempt)

Figure C-3

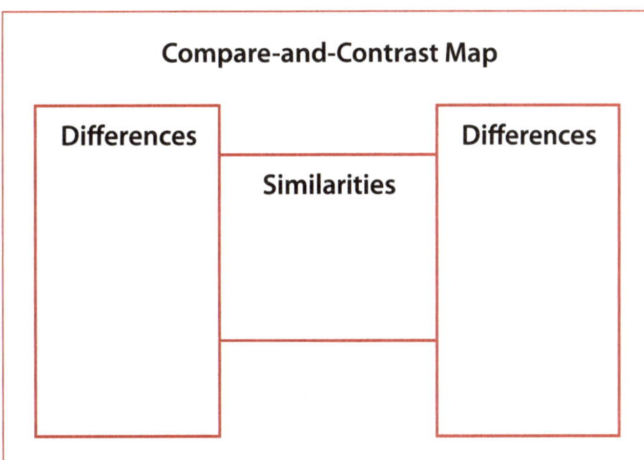

Figure C-4

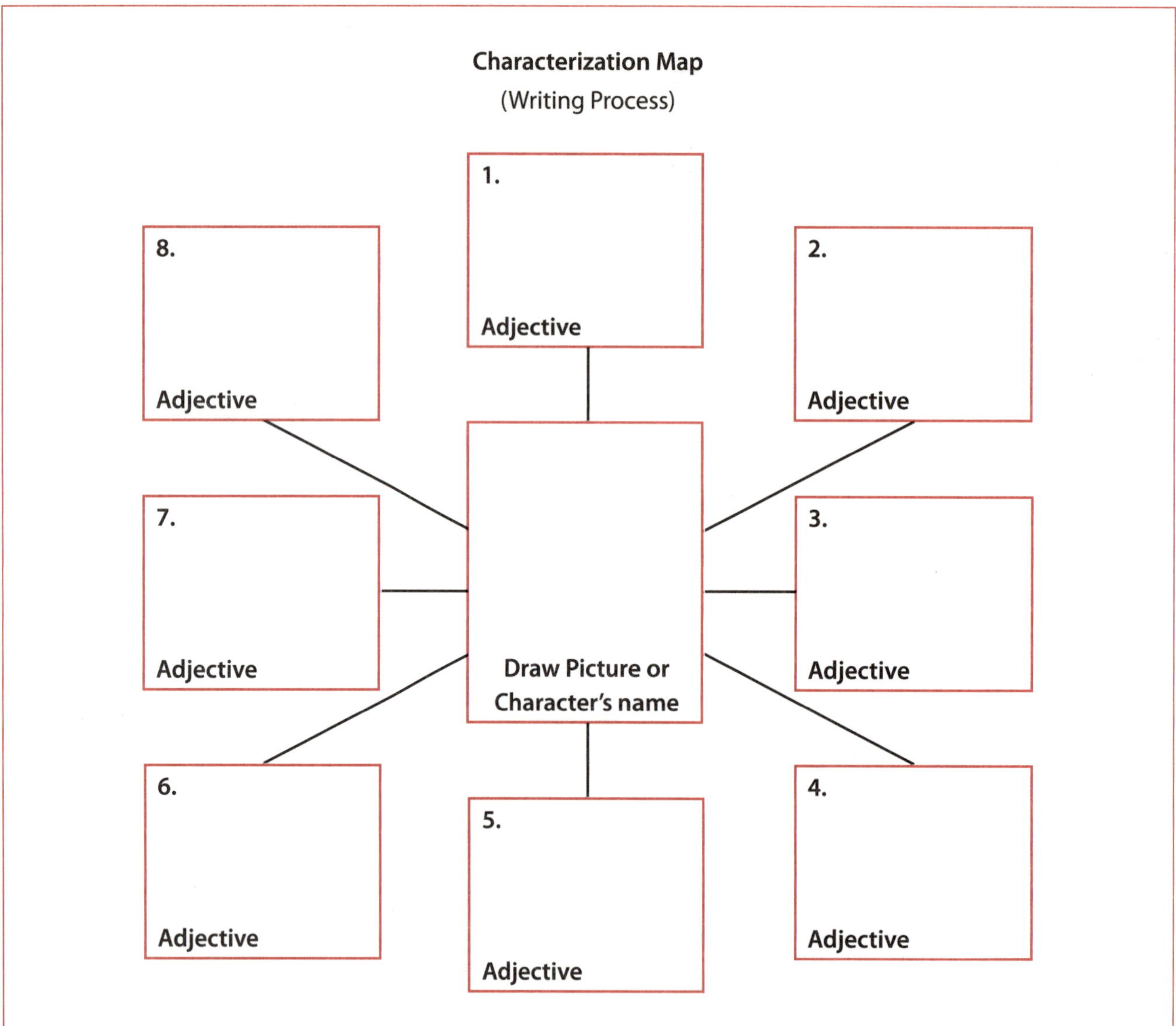
Characterization Map
(Writing Process)
1.
Adjective
2.
Adjective
3.
Adjective
4.
Adjective
5.
Adjective
6.
Adjective
7.
Adjective
8.
Adjective
Draw Picture or
Character's name

Figure C-5

Appendix D

Sentence Types

Sentence Construction	Example
Basic Sentence Forms	
1. N + is Verbing	The baby is sleeping.
2. N + is Verbing + N	The dog is eating the bone.
3. N + can V + N	The boy can fix the car.
4. N + is + Preposition	The cat is in the house.
5. N + is + Adjective	The soup is hot.
6. N + V singular + N	The clown rides the horse.
Prepositions	
7. N + is Verbing + Preposition	The boy is swimming in the water.
8. N + is Verbing + N + Preposition	The girl is riding the bike in the street.
9. N + has + N	The baby has the cracker.
10. N + has + N + Preposition	The lady has a flower in her hand.
Questions	
11. Who + is doing + N	Who is reading the newspaper?
12. Who + is doing + Preposition	Who is sitting in the chair?
13. Who + is + Preposition	Who is in the tree?
14. Who + has + N	Who has the ball?
15. Who + has + N + Preposition	Who has the money in his hand?
16. Is + N + Verbing + N	Is the boy kicking the ball?
17. Is + N + Adjective	Is the car blue?
18. Can + N + V + N	Can the girl eat the banana?
19. What + is + N + Verbing	What is the boy drinking?
20. Wh- + is + N + Verbing + N	Where/When/Why/How is the boy reading the book?
21. Which + N + is + N + Verbing	Which cat is the girl petting?
Negatives	
22. N + is + not + Verbing + N	The baby is not drinking milk.
23. N + is + not + Preposition	The book is not on the table.
24. N + is + not + Adjective	The car is not blue.
25. N + can + not + V + N	The girl cannot see the movie.
Plurals	
26. N + is Verbing + N singular/N plural	The boy is reading the book. The boy is reading the books.
27. N singular/N plural + is/are Verbing	The boy is running. The boys are running.

(continues)

Sentence Construction	Example
Pronouns	
28. He/She/It + is Verbing + N	He is climbing the tree.
29. I + am Verbing + N	I am feeding the dog.
30. We/You/They + are Verbing + N	We are feeding the dog.
31. N + is Verbing + me/him/her/it/them/us	The cat is scratching her.
Past Tense	
32. N + Verb + ed + N	The clown popped the balloon.
33. N + Verb + ed + Preposition	The cowboy jumped on the horse.
34. N/N plural + was/were Verbing + N/ N plural	The girl was playing the piano. The girls were playing the pianos.
35. N + had + N	The baby had a toy.
36. Who + Verb + ed + N	Who kicked the ball?
Future Tense	
37. N + will + V + N	The man will fix the car.
38. N + will be + Preposition/Adjective	The cat will be under the chair. The clown will be funny.
39. N + will be + Verbing + N	The girl will be running a race.
40. N + will have + N	The boy will have a sandwich.
41. N + will + not + V + N	The horse will not drink the water.
42. Will + N + V + N	Will the kitten scratch the child?
Adjectives	
43. N + is Verbing + Adjective + N	The girl is playing the blue drum.
44. N + is Verbing + Adjective + N + Preposition	The clown is riding the black horse inside the tent.
45. Adjective + N + is Verbing + N	The blue bird is eating the seed.
46. Adjective + N + is Verbing + N + Preposition	The red car is racing the truck on the tracks.

Appendix E

Purposes for Writing

Most writing takes four purposeful forms:

- Narrative
- Descriptive
- Expository
- Persuasive

What Is Narrative Writing?

A narrative is a story. It contains specific elements that work together to create interest for not only the author but also the reader. A narrative encourages readers to feel that they are a part of the story. The writer attempts to help readers feel as if they are hearing the story directly so that they experience what the characters are doing or what is being done to them. Narratives have plots to make readers wonder what will happen next. They contain conflict and dilemmas, and the resolution is important to the readers. Narratives have vivid settings that capture the imagination. Most narratives have themes, such as friendship, growing up, and survival, that make readers think about the story and its purpose long after they have finished the story. Myths, legends, fables, and other made-up stories are fiction. Authors use narrative writing techniques to tell these tales.

What Is Descriptive Writing?

Descriptive writing describes people, events, places, or objects. After planning the description, the writer uses appropriate paragraph form to compose the description. That is, the writer composes a topic sentence that will introduce the person, place, or item to be described and then provides details. The writer attempts to help readers feel that they can see, feel, hear, or taste the thing they are reading about. Writers use specific details and precise word choices. Descriptive writing includes material such as character sketches, directions to a location, and descriptions of an event (e.g., roasting marshmallows, descriptions of a room).

What Is Expository Writing?

Expository writing instructs or informs. Expository writing is nonfiction that explains and describes a process or presents facts, details, and background information about past events and discoveries. Expository is the most common form of writing and reading assigned in school. Science projects, research papers for history, and mathematical word problems are a few examples. Students often take tests that require them to write summaries, journal entries, directions, memoirs, or informational articles. In each of these, students must do expository writing. Students must identify and stay on the topic; develop the topic with simple facts, details, examples, and explanations; and exclude extraneous and inappropriate information.

What Is Persuasive Writing?

Persuasive writing persuades the reader to act or adopt an opinion. In the prewriting stage, writers must identify their audience and the desired effect of their writing. Persuasive writing may take the form of business letters to persuade readers to adopt a stand or provide a product, letters of recommendation to persuade a company or school to consider an applicant, and so on. Writers must show awareness of the audience's interests, beliefs, or priorities. Students also use persuasive writing when they must respond to or critique literature. Their responses must identify their own judgments about the literature and support their judgments with references to the text, other works, other authors, nonprint media, and personal knowledge.

Appendix F

Writing Frames

A framed sentence or paragraph is an outline using key or structure words with open spaces for students to supply their own words. Frames are a bridge to full-length composing for students. Frames may be provided for any sentence or writing form that students need to develop. Students have the option to complete the frames with as many words as they choose. It is important to encourage them to use rich vocabulary and enough words to make meaningful sentences. The following are examples of basic writing frames.

1. Frames for Sentence Types

When Sam ________________ his friend, he ________________ because ________________. (When Sam called his friend, he felt happy because he hadn't seen her for a long time.)

2. Frames to Develop Sequence and Logical Organization

When I got home from school, I noticed ________________.

By six o'clock, ________________.

By the time I was ready for bed, ________________.

3. Frames for Description Using the Word *Who*

I am a(n) ________________ who ________________.

(I am a girl who loves to play soccer with my friends.)

(Variation: Lincoln was the president who wrote the Gettysburg Address.)

4. Story or Book Report Frames

a. Frame for Describing Characters and Setting

(Title) ________________ is a book/story/novel that happened in/near/on (where/when) ________________. The main character is (person) ________________ who ________________. There are other important characters. There is ________________ who ________________. There is also ________________ who ________________. Finally, there is ________________ who ________________.

b. Frames for Describing the Problem or Theme

The problem begins when ________________.

The problem gets worse when ________________.

The problem is solved when ________________.

c. Frames for Expressing an Opinion About the Story or Book

Because I read this book, I realized/learned/understood ________________.

I would/would not recommend this book to anyone who ________________.

5. Frames for Older Students When Answering Word Problems

I first ask myself, Have I read this problem carefully?

I know that ________________.

I have to find out ________________.

To find my answer I can ________________.

I might get my answer by ________________.

Another way to solve it is ________________.

I got my answer when I ________________.

My answer is ________________ because ________________.

Note. Adapted from *Teaching Writing: Strategies for Improving Literacy Across the Curriculum* (2nd ed.), by D. Gess, 2006, Suffern, NY: ERA/CCR Corporation, The Write Track.

Appendix G

Fluency Facilitators

Suggestions for family and teachers for ways to help children improve their fluency:

- Convey to the child that you accept him/her, whether or not he/she stutters.
- Respond to what the child says, not how.
- Talk about stuttering with the child, making stuttering a "no big deal" topic for discussion, just as you might talk about any other topic.
- Talk about talking, even when you can't listen. Let the child know that you're interested in what he/she has to say. Tell the child you're busy right now, but you'll listen as soon as you're through. Make sure you really do get back to him/her in a short period of time and listen without doing anything else.
- As much as possible, establish a calm, relaxed atmosphere. Allow plenty of time to do things so that you don't have to rush from one thing to another.
- Speak in a relaxed, unhurried way, pausing frequently.
- Speak in short sentences with vocabulary appropriate to the child's age.
- Comment about what the child has done rather than ask lots of questions.
- When you must ask questions, ask *yes/no* questions, two-choice questions, or limited scope questions, such as "What was the best thing that happened on the field trip?" instead of "What happened on the field trip?"
- Allow the child to finish his/her thoughts before you respond. It's often easy to anticipate what the child is going to say and respond before he/she finishes. Let the child finish, pause for a short time, and then respond.
- Model and encourage good turn taking while talking. Count silently to 5 before responding as a way to slow down the rate of turn taking.
- Set aside a few minutes at a regular time each day when you can give the child your undivided attention. Let the child direct you in the activities and choose whether he/she talks or not. When you talk, use slow, easy speech with plenty of pauses. Allow and accept periods of silence.
- Praise, compliment, and thank the child frequently.
- Let the child own the problem of stuttering. Allow the child to handle speaking situations and show confidence in his/her ability to speak by not letting the child avoid speaking situations.
- Be an active part of the child's fluency intervention. Learn the tools or techniques the child uses to control his/her stuttering.
- There are many things family and teachers can do to help children who stutter speak more easily and fluently. The most important of these is to learn more about stuttering. A good place to start this learning process is with some of the booklets and videos by the Stuttering Foundation of America at this address:

  Suite 603
  P.O. Box 11749
  Memphis, TN 38111-0749
  1-800-992-9392
  www.stutteringhelp.org/
  stutter@stutteringhelp.org

Note. Printed with permission. Valerie Johnston, M.S., CCC-SLP, 2016, www.overtonspeech.net.

Appendix H

Correlation With Common Core State Standards

This figure was designed for speech–language pathologists (SLPs) and other professionals who wish to find goals and objectives within *The SLP's IEP Companion* that correlate with Common Core State Standards (CCSS) for English Language Arts. The CCSS are organized by strands. The following CCSS strands correlate with IEP goals and objectives:

- Reading: Literature (RL)
- Reading: Informational Text (RI)
- Reading: Foundational Skills (RF)
- Writing (W)
- Speaking and Listening (SL)
- Language (L)
- History/Social Studies (RH)
- Anchor Standards for Reading (CCRA)

To use the chart to teach multiple goals and objectives within a single strand, locate the strand in the top row. Bullets within the strand column indicate the units and sections containing goals and objectives that correlate with the strand.

To address a particular standard, find the strand that the standard falls within. For example, the following standard is within the Language strand: "Use personal, possessive, and indefinite pronouns (e.g., I, me, my; they, them, their, anyone, everything)" (CCSS.ELA-LITERACY.L.1.1.D). The letter or letters just following CCSS .ELA-LITERACY, in this case L for Language, is the strand.

CCSS.ELA-Literacy Strands

Unit	Section	Page	RL Reading: Literature	RI Reading: Informational Text	RF Reading: Foundational Skills	W Writing	SL Speaking and Listening	L Language
1	**Pragmatics**							
1	Conversational Acts in School-Age Children and Adolescents						•	
1	Classroom Communication Skills		•			•	•	
1	Classroom Social Survival Skills						•	
1	Narrative Discourse		•				•	
2	**Vocabulary and Meaning**							
2	Labels and Categories							•
2	Action and Function Concepts: Verbs							•
2	Quality Concepts: Adjectives							•
2	Position and Time Concepts: Prepositions					•		•
2	Answering Questions			•		•	•	
2	Formulating Definitions							•
2	Comparing and Contrasting Meanings							•
2	Antonyms							•
2	Synonyms							•
2	Multiple-Meaning Words							•
2	Word Relationships					•		•
2	Verbal Analogies							•
2	Figurative Language							•
2	Inferences, Predictions, and Outcomes		•					

(continues)

CCSS.ELA-Literacy Strands

Unit	Section	Page	RL Reading: Literature	RI Reading: Informational Text	RF Reading: Foundational Skills	W Writing	SL Speaking and Listening	L Language
3	**Syntax and Morphology**							
3	Negatives							•
3	Asking *Wh-* Questions		•	•			•	•
3	Asking *Yes/No* Questions		•	•			•	
3	Pronouns				•			•
3	Plural Nouns							•
3	Copular (Linking) and Auxiliary (Helping) Verbs							•
3	Possessive Nouns				•			•
3	Comparatives and Superlatives							•
3	Past Tense Verbs							•
3	Third Person Verbs							•
3	Future Tense Verbs							•
3	Articles				•			•
3	Conjunctions and Transition Words					•		•
3	Modal Auxiliaries							•
3	Complex Sentences							•
3	Passive Sentences							•
4	**Critical Thinking for Language and Communication**							
4	Recalling Information From Short- and Long-Term Memory					•		
4	Making Sense of Information Gathered						•	
4	Applying and Evaluating Information in New Situations						•	

(continues)

Unit	Section	Page	RL Reading: Literature	RI Reading: Informational Text	RF Reading: Foundational Skills	W Writing	SL Speaking and Listening	L Language
6	**Listening**							
6	Auditory Discrimination				•			
6	Listening to Evaluate a Message						•	
7	**Literacy: Reading**							
7	Reading Readiness: Age 3 Months to Kindergarten		•		•			
7	Phonological Awareness: PreK–Grade 1				•			
7	Reading Accuracy: Grades 1–5				•			
7	Reading Fluency: Grades 1–12				•			
7	Reading Comprehension of Literature: Grades 1–3		•					
7	Reading Comprehension of Literature: Grades 4–8		•					
7	Reading Comprehension of Informational Text: Grades 4–8			•				
8	**Literacy: Writing**							
8	Writing Mechanics: Grades K–7							•
8	Writing With Appropriate Form and Style: Grades 3–6					•		•
8	Writing to Communicate: Grades 1–8					•		
8	Writing Process: Grades 1–8					•		

About the Authors

Carolyn C. Wilson, MS, CCC-SLP, is a speech–language pathologist who has specialized in providing evaluations and intervention for children and adolescents with language, reading, or social language disorders. She has authored or coauthored a number of clinical books and practical therapy programs in these areas. Carolyn began her career in 1975 in the public schools. Later she served on the faculty of the Department of Communication Sciences and Disorders at Texas Christian University in Fort Worth, Texas, where she was an instructor, clinical supervisor, and clinic coordinator at the TCU Miller Speech and Hearing Clinic. She has been in private practice in Fort Worth since 1991.

Janet R. Lanza, MS, CCC-SLP, is a speech–language pathologist who has worked in public schools, private practice, and a university clinic in Texas since 1976. She was on the faculty of the Department of Communication Sciences and Disorders at Texas Christian University in Fort Worth, Texas, for 25 years. At the TCU Miller Speech and Hearing Clinic, Janet was an instructor and clinical supervisor for classroom settings of preschool children with a variety of communication disorders. She has coauthored numerous products that center on practical therapy ideas for young children and has presented nationally and internationally on that topic. Janet retired from TCU in 2014.